YOGA SUTRA

Raise Mindfulness To Discover The Light Of Your Soul

© Copyright 2019 by Mahatma Pattabhi

All rights reserved.

This document is geared towards providing exact and reliable information with regards to the topic and issue covered. The publication is sold with the idea that the publisher is not required to render accounting, officially permitted, or otherwise, qualified services. If advice is necessary, legal or professional, a practiced individual in the profession should be ordered.

- From a Declaration of Principles which was accepted and approved equally by a Committee of the American Bar Association and a Committee of Publishers and Associations.

In no way is it legal to reproduce, duplicate, or transmit any part of this document in either electronic means or in printed format. Recording of this publication is strictly prohibited and any storage of this document is not allowed unless with written permission from the publisher. All rights reserved.

The information provided herein is stated to be truthful and consistent, in that any liability, in terms of inattention or otherwise, by any usage or abuse of any policies, processes, or directions contained within is the solitary and utter responsibility of the recipient reader. Under no circumstances will any legal responsibility or blame be held against the publisher for any reparation, damages, or monetary loss due to the information herein, either directly or indirectly.

Respective authors own all copyrights not held by the publisher.

The information herein is offered for informational purposes solely, and is universal as so. The presentation of the information is without contract or any type of guarantee assurance.

The trademarks that are used are without any consent, and the publication of the trademark is without permission or backing by the trademark owner. All trademarks and brands within this book are for clarifying purposes only and are the owned by the owners themselves, not affiliated with this document.

TABLE OF CONTENTS

Introduction 1
Chapter One: Samadhi Pada 7
Chapter Two: Sadhana Pada 42
Chapter Three: Vibhuti Pada 74
Chapter Four: Kaivalya Pada 106
Conclusion 139

INTRODUCTION

Who would not want to keep their body healthy and fit? There are several diet and fitness programs in various countries that loop around. But can you believe any of them until you actually try it out? The reaction to that is' no!' Okay, what if there's a way of life that will encourage you to be versatile, increase your power of focus, relax your mind and body, physically strengthen you? You would think there might not be such a program of exercise that will give us all this in one go.

The yoga practice has always been passed down from student to instructor. Over thousands of years this experience has grown and changed, evolving ever so gradually into what we today call "yoga." Because these concepts were often kept secret and guarded, much of the yoga remained hidden in secrecy until quite recently.

Although there is no direct evidence, however, some researchers believe that yoga has been in existence since the ancient times and is more than 10,000 years old. It is assumed that this was done in Northern India's Indus-Sarasvati area.

Some of the earliest yoga evidence has been found on artefacts dating back to 3000 B.C. In the River Indus region, a team of archeologists under Sir Mortimer Wheeler found many artefacts depicting advanced yoga poses. Sir John Marshall discovered another artefact found in this area. The Pashupati is believed to be the Hindu god Shiva sitting in the place of the yogic "Lotus."

There are several texts relating to yoga as well as artefacts. The Rig-Veda, for example, an ancient Classical Indian collection of Vedic Sanskrit hymns, dates from 1700-1100 B.C.

There are also multiple references to Yoga in several Upanishads, or ancient Vedic teachings. This includes the famous Bhagavad-Gita. The Gita is a book from the Hindu chapter 700. In this verse, Lord Krishna talks, among other things, to Prince Arjuna about his duties as a warrior. Krishna also speaks lengthily about Yoga. The yoga spoken of in the Gita doesn't resemble the yoga we know today. Yoga here applies instead to a spiritual and mystical collection of minds like harmony, serenity and self-control.

In 1893 Swami Vivekananda spoke about Hindu ism and yoga at the Parliament of Religions. This speech has been widely recognized as one of the first Western introduction of yoga.

Modern Times Yoga came about with the birth of a man named Sri Tirumalai Krishnamachary in 1888. Thus, Krishnamacharya was known as the "father of modern yoga." He taught many now famous students of yoga: B.K.S. Iyengar, T.K.V. Desikachar and Pattabhi Jois.

B.K.S. Iyengar was born in 1918 and has become one of the most famous yoga teachers in the modern world. He published the landmark book "Light on Yoga" in 1966 which popularized yoga worldwide.

Demand for yoga exploded in the West in the 1960's. At the moment, the U.S. was experiencing a kind of spiritual change, and people increasingly turned to the Eastern philosophies as a way to achieve peace and happiness.

Dr. Dean Ornish brought meditation and physical health together in the 1980's when he recommended yoga practice to maintain a strong and healthy heart.

In the Western World today's yoga tends to focus mostly on the physical benefits of its practice. Hundreds of yoga studios literally exist all over the world. A Yoga Journal survey in 2008 found that 15.8 million people practice yoga in the US. That number grows every day as yoga increasingly becomes one of the most popular forms of exercise in the West.

When we hear the term "yoga" it brings to mind for most people the image of a model on the cover of a yoga magazine, in a seemingly weird posture that would be nearly impossible for an ordinary person to get into. Yoga is widely practiced as an exercise that helps to improve physical fitness, and sometimes as a way of managing stress. There is a growing awareness that it can be used effectively in the treatment of a variety of ailments, including hypertension, diabetes, heart conditions etc. Those who have been practicing yoga for some time can testify to the physical and physiological benefits the practice brings.

Although all of the above attributes are undoubtedly beneficial, most people are unaware of the true meaning and purpose of yoga, which is "the ability to control mind fluctuations." Sage Patanjali provided us with this brief and concise description, more than three thousand years ago. Patanjali has given a very scientific and realistic explanation of the yoga theory and practice in his Sutras.

Yoga has an illustrious and rich history. The basics are rooted in tradition and stories that provide you with clear and simple guidance for a safe and spiritual life. Many people are drawn to the philosophy of yoga and also to the more physical aspects of yoga.

Have you learnt about Patanjali from your Yoga Teacher? Or use the terms Yoga Sutra, Yama and Niyamas and ask what does that have to do with Yoga? Are you aware that yoga is more than 5,000 years old, and originally practiced by monks and seers as a way to help them connect more deeply with the divine?

The origins of yoga can be traced back to the Indus Valley Civilization which flourished in the Indus River Basin (mature era 2600-1900 BCE). This region covers most of Pakistan and stretches into parts of modern India. Many individuals discovered during the Indus Valley Civilization (c.3300-1700 BC) series of human figures in yoga postures or meditation, which indicate that yoga was practiced then.

The word ' yoga' comes from the language of Sanskrit, which means union. There are many yoga schools, but the aim is always the same, in each individual and the divine, to achieve union, complete harmony between body, mind and spirit traditionally.

In today's modern era, many students view yoga purely as a form of physical exercise and fail to realize that a deep and long-standing philosophical history and tradition lies behind the physical exercises.

The "mind" aspect of Yoga is often denied in meditation practice. It goes deeper than this though, and has its roots steeped in yogic tradition. The philosophical side of yoga is to run alongside your practice of asanas and meditation. Yoga philosophy offers you a better understanding of the relationship that exists between your soul, body and mind.

The Patanjali Yoga Sutra is one of the most popular texts about the philosophy of yoga. Widely influenced by the great Indian sage Patanjali, the first introduction to philosophy by most modern-day yoga students is by their introduction to the Yamas and Niyamas or by hearing the words "the Eight Limbs of Yoga."

Many people today practice what is called Hatha Yoga, which includes physical postures (asanas) and some methods for breathing (pranayama). Nevertheless, in order to develop a fully integrated practice and attain the ultimate goals of mind control, one must in some way include all the eight limbs in their routine.

Overview of Yoga Sutra

The Yoga Sutras is one of six philosophical branches in Hindu philosophy schools and a very important milestone in the history of yoga. It is a collection of 195 aphorisms (sutras), short, tight phrases designed to memorize easily. Though short, it is a highly important work that is as essential to the practice of yoga today. The sutras are divided into four chapters (pada) as follows: A brief overview of the four chapters of the Yoga Sutras is given below.

- Samadhi Pada: This introductory chapter contains 51 sutras focusing on meaning, practice, challenges, approaches to yoga practice, and achieving higher states of consciousness that we often refer to as "meditative absorption."

- Sadhana Pada: The second chapter contains 55 sutras focusing on gaining and retaining mental focus. Sadhana Pada offers the reader information on how to maintain states of concentration (mindfulness), rather than live in a distracted state.

- Vibhuti Pada: The third chapter includes 55 sutras and is a guide to the simultaneous focus (dharana), meditation (dhyana), and communion (samadhi) practice combined. The "tying together" concept is a technique called "samyama" which is a technique for having a more in-depth emphasis.

- Kaivalya Pada: This last chapter contains 34 sutras which reveal Yoga's primary goals. The keys to spiritual liberty, outlined within the Kaivalya Pada, are used to master one's mind, develop a perception of pure clarity and be free from attachment.

CHAPTER ONE
SAMADHI PADA

---

1. atha yoganushasanam

Not later, not quite soon: it has to be now.

If we want to understand the principles of Yoga, our minds cannot be bogged or worried about the future. With all other worries being at least temporarily put aside, our minds are at the moment free. In all areas of learning, but especially in spiritual matters, the ability to focus attention is an important requirement which contains subtle philosophical observations.

2. yogashchittavrittinirodhah

This is the core of Raja Yoga. Every single word has a heavy meaning. This sutra alone could form the basis of meditation and practice throughout life.

In Sanskrit, the four words that comprise this sutra are: Yogas, chitta, vritti and nirodha.

Yoga, the word "yoga" has become so much a part of our everyday language that we take it for granted with the believe that we understand its significance. Derived from the root, yuj, this refers to the act of yoking. It refers to the harnessing of animals into carts for their use. It is the origin from which we derive the English word "yoke." Chitta comes from the meaning, "to experience, to learn, to observe." Translated throughout this text as "thinking" or "mind-stuff," this refers to the entirety of the mind: being aware, subconscious and unconscious.

The chitta is neither a separate part of Prakriti, nor a Purusha counterpart. It is the reflection of purusha on Prakriti consciousness. As such, chitta is a way of understanding the relationship between the Purusha (the Seer) and Prakriti (the seen)

Vritti: literally meaning whirling, spinning, rotating, moving forward. It is a colorful term, suggesting an incessant and perhaps dizzying movement. A vritti is not a pure thought; it is the behavior that occurs in the mind to form conceptions from individual thoughts. This happens on both the conscious and subconscious levels of the mind.

Nirodha is used for both process and state denotation. It is often translated into containment, termination, restraint, repression, avoidance, regulation, and inhibition. Nirodha is usually associated with practices to quiet the mind— making it quiet, clear, and focused where the difficulty of understanding becomes less compounded.

Nonetheless, the capacity of nirodha to still vrittis behavior is not due to physical coercion, but rather to a mechanism of selective focus: to shift and retain attention to one object or concept. Other vrittis are naturally restrained from consciousness during this process, breaking the usual routine of vritti activity. It frees the mind from the usual perception patterns which obscure the true nature of life and self. In a fresh new light, the mind begins to perceive everything, to see things as they are. That is why activities such as worship, meditation, selfless service and research, which also rely on selective attention, contribute to the vrittis ' grip on the mind being released.

3. tada drashtuh svaroope avasthanam

The Seer (Self) then abides in His own nature.

The Seer has nothing but the power of seeing things through the mind. "Seer is another way of referring to the Purusha: pure consciousness; unchanging, unconditional awareness.

The Seer, though always present as our True Self, seems to appear and vanish because of frequent movements of the mind. What is being suggested here is that when the mind becomes restless the Seer will no longer be a visitor, rather it will come with periods of mental stillness and leave.

The last two sutras present the basic theoretical core of Raja Yoga; that all traces of ignorance disappear in a perfectly still, clear mind, and the person experiences him or herself as pure, eternal, as well as unbounded awareness.

You were probably asked at some stage during your grade-school years to memorize a poem to read the next day. What did you say if you were perfectly aware of that? "I know it from heart." Not from head, mind or brain, but from heart. Heart implies the mind as a whole, something deeper and more stable than the usual apparatus of thought. Keeping a pure heart is keeping a healthy, steady mind -

a nirodha state. The consequence of that innocence is the fact that we are going to see God. There is no implied choice. If your heart is pure, you're going to see God; no ifs, nor buts.

4. vrittisaroopyam itaratra

At other times, the seer (appearing to be the Self) assumes the forms of the mental changes.

This describes the habit of clinging to individuality: the mental activity identifying ego. The whirlpool of mental change (vrittis) has a way to captivate our attention. It's such a captivating drama that in the theatrics we lose ourselves (and Self). We forget we're truly witnesses of the play.

The misidentification process is unspeakably innocent. For starters, if we look in a mirror at our reflection, we think that we are the body. "I'm tall." "I'm thin." "I'm male." "I'm sick." We say different statements when we identify with the mind's content. "I'm a physics professor." "I'm a doctor." "I'm happy." "I'm sad." Yet the Self has not changed. It's the Mind-mirror reflection of the Self that shifts

5. vrittayah pangchatayyah klishta aklishtah

There are five types of behavioral changes which are either painful or painless.

By category

The divisions consist of the five primary tasks performed by the mind while engaged in everyday life (see sutra 1.6 for the list).

By effect

Mental behavior is essentially guided by a dualist concept. The focus of the mind typically flows in one of two directions: towards tasks which are pleasurable or distant from those which cause pain.

Note the words used in this sutra: "painful or painless." We mistakenly (sometimes subconsciously) think that there is a philosophy or set of spiritual exercises which will put an end to the suffering and bring pleasure. We believe this because we forget that in reality, the pleasure we seek is who we already are. And although it is true that vritti activity has only two effects, it is not pain and enjoyment. The reality is that vritti behavior can either mask our true nature's happiness, or leave that happiness undisturbed.

Clarity, discernment, and selflessness are characteristics of the flow toward the painless. That stream of thought leads to the dissolution of ignorance. On the other hand, ignorance affects mental behaviors that cause suffering, and helps to maintain its power and influence. These two basic movements are like whirlpools, gaining momentum or losing momentum according to the person's thoughts and actions.

6. pramannaviparyayavikalpanidrasmritayah

These behavioral changes are right knowledge, confusion, conceptualisation, sleep and memory.

This sutra tells you what the vrittis "look like." Having a good description of how individuals look or act is helpful if we want to catch thieves. If our aim is to achieve nirodha in the mind over the vrittis, a description of them would be very useful.

One can divide these five vrittis into three groups. The first is about the way we collect information, regardless of whether it is valid or invalid. The second is the opposite of data gathering i.e. — thinking of nothing and its consequence, this state is what we call sleeping. It is how the mind reaches a state of profound rest. The third is memory, which allows for learning through retaining experiences and giving continuity to life.

Sleep, memories, and knowledge — right or wrong— all these is in the realm of mental modifications, and therefore should ultimately come under our mastery, according to Sri Patanjali.

7. pratyakshanumanagamah pramanani

The origins of right knowledge are direct observation, inference, and authoritative testimony.

Our understanding of life is built on the basis of the knowledge that we gain throughout life. But that information can only be trusted if it is obtained by valid means.

Knowledge obtained by real perception can be viewed as factual, meaning it is consistent with the facts themselves. Not only is experience the best teacher; it is actually the only teacher. Even reading a book or taking a class is profiting from the experience of somebody else. We can learn about fire that it generates heat and can either be put to harmful or positive uses. It could all be important, but if our fire experience is limited to words on a page, this remains a reality outside of our knowledge. We can't say we know what kind of fire is. But when we place our finger near the flame, we know it can burn our flesh; and we will understand its value after cooking food over a fire.

Inference is mainly a function of the mind's (buddhi) discriminative faculties, which depends on previously acquired awareness. It requires that we know at least some of the characteristics of the inferred object, and can relate those characteristics to the object correctly. The classic example is that when we see smoke, fire can be assumed, because one of the features of fire is that it is accompanied by smoke.

Authoritative testimony (Agama), literally, meaning "going to a source," expert advice and instruction from scriptures and spiritual adherents or learned persons.

The direct experience of the sages, saints, prophets, and spiritual leaders is a reliable source of knowledge, as it is knowledge that has proven its value over time to countless seekers. It should also be knowledge that the individual has the potential to be verified through his or her own direct perception. Once we drive on the roads by ourselves, we will check the authenticity of the road maps in our guidebook.

8. viparyayo mithyajnanam atadroopapratishtham

Misperception takes place when knowing something is not based on its true form.

Viparyaya is the term translated as misperception. The origins of the word provide a hint about what it is, and how it happens.

Viparyaya is from I "moving, flowing," with vi, "asunder, down," and pari, "about," giving Viparyaya, "flowing away or around." Misperception happens when the mind misses the point and flows away from or around the facts when it draws a conclusion about an event.

Remember how this concept of misperception is almost the direct opposite of nirodha — holding steady focus from the mind. The implication is that when the mind is missing a firm concentration, conclusions can be flawed. Misperception is rooted in problems that occur during the perception act or the inference process. It may be that the information transmitted by the senses is insufficient, the reasoning is wrong, irrelevant knowledge is introduced or the memory does not contain evidence related to the perceived object. The effect of misperception is that mental experiences (vrittis) that do not correlate to actual facts are processed as true knowledge and regarded as such.

9. shabdajnaananupati vastushoonyo vikalpah

Conceptualization is knowledge which is based on language alone, independent of any external object.

Across different ways, the mind builds our understanding of life. Knowledge born of conceptualization is based solely on language: on our familiarity with words and the knowledge that words symbolize. Conceptualization is the development of abstract perceptions from the incessant dialogs of the mind within. Perhaps it is the most influential maker of our notions about truth. Consider how many of our ideas about existence are formed from or based on what we hear in conversations and through novels, newspapers, films, television shows, and lyrics for a moment.

The subconscious weaves experiences in conceptualisation by incorporating memory and language in different creative ways. It is important to note that the information gained by conceptualisation may or may not be right. Consider the adage, "Love is blind," for example, a proposal that has no perceptible object we can connect to. It is a reality built of words alone which can indeed reflect a reality. First, we come across the saying, "God is love." Again, the senses don't detect any thing, and once again— using only words — we treat these words as reality. In a poetic way, these two sayings echo personal feelings which are true and which can become building blocks of our worldview.

10. abhavapratyayalambana vrittirnidra

Sleep is that mental modification that depends upon the thought of nothingness.

It applies to the sleeping without dreaming. It is the condition in which all other vrittis, except that of nothingness, are suspended; the fact that we recall sleeping shows that the pure lack of mental activity is not sleep. We only know what we experience.

While deep sleep offers much-needed healing rest for the body, the deeper and subtler role of sleep is mind rejuvenation. The body may get some recovery in other ways, though it needs rest so it can regenerate. For the advanced yogi, deep meditation states provide both body and mind with profound rest and rejuvenation.

11. anubhootavishayasanpramoshah smritih

Memory is the recollection of the events encountered.

As vrittis, all interactions have an effect on the mind. After a while, the vrittis become subtler and sink to the bottom of the mental lake, where they become samskaras: impressions of subconsciousness. Samskaras may lie dormant and not affect us, become active at a subconscious level and influence our conscious mental states, or be stimulated and return as memory to the surface of the mental lake.

This sutra has an association with the previous one. Dreams are memories that hold their own in sleep. These memories can be presented in symbolic form and are therefore often not recognized as such.

Memory is the only one of the five waves of thought concerned with the past. We couldn't learn from experience, without it.

12. abhyasavairagyabhyan tannirodhah

Practice and nonattachment restrict the mental modifications.

This two-pronged approach typifies a principle employed by holistic practitioners in health care. While adequate treatment is prescribed for the present complaint, measures are also suggested to strengthen resistance to future occurrences. Practice is analogous to prevention, and non-attachment to treatment. To Yoga success, both practice and non-attachment are important. These are complementary approaches which enable the mind to become clearer, quieter and stronger.

Unattached behavior will lead to a super-inflated ego that enjoys using power to fulfill self-interest regardless of the consequences. In Hindu mythology, many demons were advanced yogis who fell from the path of righteousness when they succumbed to a tragic flaw, usually a burning craving. On the other hand, true non-attachment may never really dawn without the intensity and mental insight obtained from the practice. The mind may be falling into apathy, instead. This pseudo nonattachment can provide the scared individual with a safe haven— a moral refuge where they can disappear and escape burdens and obligations. If fears remain untouched, inherent potential remains unfathomable. We become Clark Kent, never knowing that Superman is inside. It is practice that we are mining our untapped internal resources.

13. tatra sthitau yatno abhyasah

Striving for steadiness is practice of these two.

"Effort towards steadiness" refers to focusing and quieting the mind in meditation, cultivating regularity, and developing an unwavering awareness of the activities of the mind (especially the limiting and harmful effect of the ego). Practice is, in the most general sense, the ongoing effort to remain within the flow (habit) of mental activity which leads to the dissolution of ignorance.

The practices described in the Yoga Sutras fall into the following categories:

- Asana and pranayama physical activities
- Meditation (dharana, dhyana, samadhi)
- Devotion to God or self-surrender (Ishwara Pranidhana)
- Knowing and acknowledging suffering as a healing aid (tapas)
- Discriminatory discernment (viveka)
- Practice (svadhyaya) Good results in all of these practices.

14. sa tu dirghakalanairantaryasatkarasevito dridha - bhoomih

Practice becomes firmly grounded when well attended to for a long time, without break, and with enthusiasm.

What is a "solidly based" practice, and why is it a desirable state? A strongly rooted activity is one which occurs daily without pressure or grudging participation. It has sense, motivation and emphasis. It is a joyful habit which accompanies practitioners throughout their lives and becomes the unbroken thread which guides them to self-realization.

A deeply rooted practice is not merely an established pattern of spiritual activities but an awaited link period to deeper self-levels. It is a time of rising identification with our True Self, of spiritual exploration and nurturance. In reality, times are periods of integration and rising wholeness. This realistic vision is the ideal and is attainable by anyone who follows the advice given in this sutra.

Achieving a deeply rooted practice marks an important stage in spiritual pursuits: it's the change from "doing yoga" to becoming a natural expression of who we are. Practices are no longer activities outside of us — techniques or observances added to our everyday lives. Practices like eating and sleeping become as important to our life experience.

15. drishtanushravikavishayavitrishnnasy vashikara samjna vairagyam

Nonattachment is the expression of self-mastery in one who is free to desire things that are seen or heard about.

Nonattachment, vairagya, literally means "without colour." It is the ability to keep the distortions of selfish motives and intent out of all relationships, actions and learning processes.

Selfish desires are the mind's typical motivating forces, pulling it toward the pleasure hoped for or away from the pain dread. Egoistic impulses, however, are not the correct mode of functioning for those interested in self-realization, since they are focused on relieving the pain of addiction and not on what is emotionally, psychologically, socially or spiritually advantageous. Seekers are called upon to develop another reason for their actions: nonattachment.

Nonattachment arises when the mind voluntarily changes its underlying motivations from selfish to selfless, from the search for sense satisfaction to the search for a peaceful experience that transcends external conditions. Selfless impulses slowly free the mind from the grasp of sense-motivated behavior and open it up to the Purusha's mighty power.

16. tatparan purushakhyatergunnavaitrishnyam

Because of the Purusha realization, even when the gunas (constituents of Nature) are not thirsty, that is supreme nonattachment.

In Nature, there are three gunas or qualities: sattwa, brightness, or balance; rajas, restlessness, or activity; and tamas, dullness, or inertia. Every generated material (including the mind) is composed of these three qualities. In a given entity, the mix of gunas varies and is not constant, with their interactions accounting for changes in the matter. There is absolutely nothing the experienced yogi longs for in Nature (see sutras 2.18 and 2.19 for more on the gunas).

This stage of nonattachment is the natural result of the process started in the previous sutra, which explained vairagya as a "manifestation of self-mastery," a state requiring effort and analysis. When the mind desires an inappropriate thing, you say, "No," to the mind, and it stays away. Even though you may be able to free yourself from new temptations, subtle impressions are still stored in the mind— memories that will tempt you. The cravings resulting from subtle impressions aren't erased easily. But you don't even worry about adding on this higher level of nonattachment. Supreme nonattachment is based on having such a good, rewarding and compelling inner experience that there is nothing out there that can compete with it. Through life, the yogi is completely free of cravings for anything.

17. vitarkavicharanandasmitaroopanugamat sanprajnatah

Cognitive samadhi (samprajnata) (is associated with forms and) is attended by examination, insight, joy and pure oneness.

Within Yoga, the term samadhi is usually used to refer to higher states of consciousness, a word typically translated as meditation, super-conscious mind, or absorption. Before going on to the meaning on this sutra, let's take a brief overview of the state of samadhi, since understanding the philosophy and practice of Yoga is central.

In a general sense, samadhi is a supra (above)-rational way of attaining knowledge. Samadhi is radically different from our usual method of interpretation in the sense that there are no measures of reasoning and no comparison or contrast of bits of information to achieve an understanding of the object being contemplated. Rather, knowledge gained from samadhi is simple, spontaneous, and intuitive, the result of achieving at least some meaningful measure of unity with the entity being envisaged.

Although the insights revealed in samadhi are not the product of a process of rational thought, they do not contradict, but transcend the rational. Samadhi (and the theory and practice of Yoga in general) is not a trip into an insane mental landscape in which fancy flights rule the day. But since samadhi has the power to go beyond the confines of physical senses, personal biases, and relativistic thinking processes ' inherent limitations, it completes and verifies knowledge gained through direct perception, inference, and authoritative testimony.

18. viramapratyayabhyasapoorvah sanskarashesho anyah

With the cessation of all conscious thought, noncognitive (asamprajnata) samadhi occurs i.e. only the subconscious impressions remain.

Asamprajnata: asam, "without," and prajna, "knowledge," giving "without knowledge," or, "not," and samprajnata, giving samadhi "not samprajnata" (the "other" samadhi).

Asamprajnata samadhi is noncognitive, as there are no objects to be discerned in the conscious mind; even the ego is transcended temporarily. Though the conscious mind becomes completely still, the impressions of the subconscious (samskaras) remain. Asamprajnata samadhi is the experience of the Purusha's reflection on an absolutely still, clear mind.

The steps from samprajnata to asamprajnata samadhis are:

• First you understand Nature (gross and subtle elements; mind and ego)

• Then bring it under your power

• Eventually, you conquer it by freeing the mind from all mental activity. Even when subconscious experiences remain, the yogi cannot be released from the ego until it transcends the samskaras.

Samskaras are remnants of past experiences which help to perpetuate vritti activity by preserving the ego structure. To reach the highest samadhi, nirbija samadhi, it is important to whip out even the samskaras.

19. bhavapratyayo videhaprakritilayanam

At the time of death, yogis who have not attained asamprajnata samadhi remain attached to Prakriti because of the continued existence of thoughts of becoming.

This sparsely worded sutra (the original Sanskrit is just five words) can be interpreted in several valid and useful ways, all of which demonstrate the same underlying principle: the continued existence of ignorance is what prevents the seeker from advancing into asamprajnata samadhi.

In samprajnata samadhi, the mind has penetrated itself into the foundation of matter, into the pure mind, and finally into the ego, into the sense of "I." Yet the power of denial over functioning of the mind persists. The "thinking to become" is the enduring desire to observe Prakriti embodied artifacts of meaning. The desire continues even after passing from the physical body, if not transcended in life. With the attainment of asamprajnata samadhi, the condition in which "all con-scientific thought comes to a standstill and only subconscious thoughts remain," the "thinking for becoming" ceases.

20. shraddhaviryasmritisamadhiprajnapoorvaka itaresham

To others, samadhi asamprajnata is followed by faith, courage, mindfulness, (cognitive) samadhi, and discernment.

Seekers are looking to experience the life's source, the essence of all things: God. Through prayer, worship, and meditation, they can experience sensations or thoughts that lead them to believe that what is happening is sacred, that their belief in God is being validated. But how do they know? In the above case, although it did exist, our perceptive forces could not detect hypertension. In many ways, our mind can get fooled.

21. tivrasanveganam aasannah

This samadhi comes very easily to the sharp and intent practicer.

Yoga success comes easier for those who have youth exuberance. Adolescents have a fearlessness— willingness to explore unfamiliar areas of life and live it. We believe we can accomplish any target, if we try hard enough. We know as we get older that we can't have everything we aspire for — and that's part of maturing. But we sometimes lose the willing energy of young people in that process. Of course we should look before we jump, but once the decision to jump is made, it should be done with all our heart. Seekers who dive with vigor and passion in themselves receive results faster. Success inspires and enthuses even more. If we're focused, inspired, dedicated, fearless of setbacks, and always seeking to grow and learn, we'll be making rapid progress.

22. mridumadhyadhimatratvat tatopi visheshah

The amount of time needed to succeed often depends on whether the practice is mild, moderate or severe.

The previous sutra had spoken about the practitioner's zeal. This sutra expands on the idea of intensity, the number of practices carried out and the degree to which they are integrated into everyday life. The more practices embedded in daily life, the sooner the influence of ignorance diminishes.

A mild practice describes one that is most likely irregular and lacks steady enthusiasm. Practice is limited for these students, and is considered a mandatory chore. Middle category practitioners usually find at least some time every day to fit in the practice of Yoga. We reap rewards but we remain isolated from much of their life from the rest of their lives. Zealous practicers emphasize sadhana. They remain motivated and concentrated, and are looking forward to practice times. Often, they seem to see every aspect of their lives as a growth opportunity. Practice is becoming a character trait for them.

23. eeshvarapranidhanad va

Or samadhi is achieved through devotion to God (Ishwara), with total dedication.

Up to this point, the emphasis was on activities that work directly with the changes in the mind by redirecting or sustaining attentiveness. Here, we find another path to realization of Self.

Devotion (pranid-hana), literally translated, means "placing or holding in front." It means giving prime importance to God's devotion of our time, abilities and resources. This sutra, in short, presents God's selfless love as a legitimate path to self-realization. Naturally, our minds dwell on that which we love. If we love someone in earthly relationships, we cannot stop thinking about them. We look forward to seeing them, conversing with them, meeting them and helping them. We would rather do nothing more than to be with our sweetheart. The same is true with God's love. Those who have a loving, dedicated attitude toward God will realize that nirodha's selective focus is easier to attain, and because loving is fun, it is more pleasant. Also, regularity and excitement are easier to attain (see sutra 14, on firmly grounded practice). There are obviously advantages that attend Ishwara's devotion.

Ishwara is derived from ish, "ruling or possessing," and may be considered the Supreme Ruler of Creation. It is the Purusha as experienced from within Prakriti's confines, and perceived through the ego's limits. Ishwara isn't separate from Purusha (Self), but is a way to outsource it.

24..kleshakarmavipakashayairaparamrishtah purushavishesh eeshvarah

Ishwara is the ultimate Purusha, untouched by any afflictions, acts, fruits of deeds or any inner sensations of desires.

How do we answer to God?

The sutra refers to Ishwara as the "supreme Purusha." Purusha has different meanings which include spirit, individual soul, or person. It is a word commonly used when referring to any person. We are all purushas, but Ishwara is the supreme because He/She/it is free from subconscious thoughts and not tainted by any afflictions or karma at all. Ishwara, in other words, is just like us but without ignorance and its implications. The equation read from the other side of course is that we are Ishwara, (apparently) limited by ignorance

25. tatra niratishayan sarvajntvabijam

The entire manifestation of the seed of omniscience is in Ishwara.

This underlines Ishwara's worthiness as an object of worship. This sutra can also teach us something about the relationship between finite and infinite, and function as proof of the Infinite's existence. Close your eyes, and take a circle shot. What's your opinion of it? Blackness: Blackness. Where ends the gloom? It just isn't. Make the circle taller. What's around it? More gloom. Where ends blackness? It is not over. And so forth. All thoughts, facts, conjectures and aspirations are finite realities that are projected onto Ishwara's infinite omniscient screen. One can know the small self because it appears against an omniscient context.

26. sa poorvesham   api guruh kalenanavachchhedat

Ishwara, unconditioned by time, is the teacher of even the oldest teachers.

We learned in the preceding sutra that Ishwara knows all there is to know. We are now discovering something about the nature of

Divine knowledge. This precious knowledge, like the valuables in a safe deposit box, should not be saved. It only accomplishes its destiny when it is communicated to those who lack it. Just as it is our nature to look for knowledge, sharing it is the nature of Ishwara. "Unconditioned by time" implies that the infinite storehouse of knowledge and wisdom at Ishwara is eternally present and always available. The knowledge available to yesterday's yogis remains available today, and will remain available for an infinite number of tomorrows.

For another cause, the language of this sutra is worthy of note. We are not told Ishwara is information source. Alternatively, Ishwara is described as teachers ' instructor (literally, guru). The word "guru" probably took on a meaning for students who lived in a society with a long-established tradition of gaining spiritual knowledge through a trained teacher's guidance. For them, it was possibly as common to seek guidance from a master as getting the weather report from the TV is for us.

27. tasya vachakah prannavah

Ishwara's phrase is OM, the magical message.

This sutra presents us with the mantra OM which denotes Ishwara. The word "OM" isn't mentioned in the Sanskrit. Instead, we find the term, pranavah, prana humming. OM is the hum of the Creation business: the creation, evolution, and destruction of beings and things. You can hear it in the roar of a fire, the ocean's deep rumble or the ground-shaking rush of the winds of a tornado.

Because pranavah isn't something that we can chant easily, the name is given as OM. It always vibrates within us and on many levels replays the drama of creation, evolution, and dissolution. In deep meditation, this hum can be heard when the external sound is transcended and the internal chatter is stilled.

28. tajjapastadarthabhavanam

Repeating it in a meditative way shows its importance.

Artha and bhavanam are the two key words in that sutra.

- Artha means meaning, or purpose; to point out, from the root "arth."

- The meanings of Bhavanam include meditation, thoughtfulness, disposition, feeling and mental discipline. Many branches of Hindu philosophy consider bhavana as a particular mental disposition—one in which things are done or remembered all the time. Repetition of mantra is not the mindless parroting of a sound, but an attentive and informed act set against an enthusiastic background. This requires constant mental focus and an awareness of the mantra's meaning. In this way the mantra's meaning (or purpose) will slowly unfold. This interpretation is in line with one of the basic tenets of Raja Yoga: concentrated attention results in deeper and more nuanced experiences.

Each and every repetition for keen seekers is a moment of connection with the Self, an affirmation of the Truth of their own spiritual identity, and a reminder of their intentions.

29. tatah pratyakchetanadhigamopyantarayabhavashch

The awareness turns inside out from this practice, and the distracting obstacles vanish.

When the mind "tunes in" with OM's vibration, it becomes introspective and begins to awaken to Self-knowledge. Meanwhile the distracting obstacles (see sutra 1.30), which are the product of a dispersed mind, dissolve naturally. By extension, we could claim a similar advantage for the repetition of any mantra and for the practice of meditation in general. They can be destroyed by meditation in the active state.

In Raja Yoga, this sutra presents a key theme: the activities do not carry spiritual development directly; they simply remove barriers that hinder it. Human evolution occurs naturally when that which retards its advancement is removed.

• They [accept pain as an aid for purification, study, and surrender] help us minimize obstacles and achieve samadhi.

• By the practice of the Yoga limbs, the impurities dwindle away and the light of wisdom dawns there, resulting in discriminative discernment.

• Incidental events do not cause natural evolution directly; they simply remove obstacles as a farmer does [removes obstacles in a waterway running to his field].

30.vyadhistyanasanshayapramadalasyaviratibhrantidarsha nalabdhabhoomikatvanavasthitatvani chittavikshepastentarayah

Disease, sluggishness, uncertainty, carelessness, laziness, sensuality, false perception, failure to reach firm ground, and falling from gained ground— these mental disturbances are the obstacles.

Those who have practiced Yoga for any length of time will be familiar with this list of obstacles. Each aspirant faces them on their spiritual journey at various points.

Vikshepa, translated as "distraction," means false (mind-stuff) reflection, scattering, dispersing, and shaking. Vikshepa suggests the barriers are symptoms of a lack of focus or loss. Ironically, misperception is also born out of a lack of steady mental focus (see sutra 1.8). Again, and again we see why nirodha is the cornerstone of spiritual life— the ability to attain a clear focused mind.

31..duhkhadaurmanasyanggamejayatvashvasaprashvaa vikshepasahabhuvah

The mental disturbances are followed by dis-stress, depression, body shaking and disturbed breathing.

The challenges in life do not actually appear to us as described in the preceding sutra. Not many clinicians have said, "These days I play with false perception." The challenges are like viruses. We cannot detect their existence directly in our systems. We need to continue to understand the signs. This sutra presents the main hindering symptoms.

32. tatpratishedhartham ekatattvabhyasah

Focusing on a single subject (or using one technique) is the best way to avoid obstacles and their accompaniment.

Meditation is presented in sutra 1.29 as the way to overcome obstacles; here we learn that engagement is the preventive against future occurrences. Steadiness of mind is the foundation of both therapies, manifesting in meditation as focused attention and life-long perseverance.

33. maitreekarunamuditopekshanansukhaduhkhapunyapunyavishayanan bhavanatashchittaprasadanam

The mind retains its undisturbed calmness by cultivating attitudes of friendliness toward the happy, compassion for the unhappy, delight in the virtuous, and equanimity toward the non-virtuous.

This sutra shows how in any situation, the mind can retain its peace. Sri Swami Satchidananda has referred to it as "the four locks and four keys." These are the "locks;" the puzzles or challenges which we face every day. The "keys" applied to these situations help the mind retain calmness without disturbance. The locks and keys are not prescriptions for specific actions: we are not told what to do but how to be; how to cultivate attitudes that make sure the instrument of perception (the mind) is in the best condition to make the proper assessments and choices.

34. prachchhardanavidharanabhyan va prannasya

Or the controlled exhalation or retention of the breath retains that calmness.

Mind and breath are linked. When the mind is calm, the breath is as it is. When the body gets agitated, then the mind follows. When we regulate the breath, the mind becomes clearer and quieter. We exert a strong soothing effect on the mind by slowly expanding the length of the exhalations and gradually increasing the retention of breath.

(A note of caution: breath retention is a very effective activity. It should be done only under the supervision of a qualified teacher to avoid any potential physical harm)

35. vishayavati va pravrittirutpanna manasah sthitinibandhini

Or that (undisturbed calmness) is achieved when the perception of a subtle object of sense arises, holding the mind steady.

For some seekers, the knowledge of something out of the ordinary serves as a motivation to persevere in their work.

Tradition recommends many ways to gain the awareness of implicit sensations of the senses: for example, constant attention on the tip of the nose or tongue. If your focus is intense and secure enough, you'll experience the first technique with a sweet scent and the second with a wonderful taste.

36. vishoka va jyotishmati

Or by concentrating inward on the ultimate, ever-blissful Sun.

This sutra applies to meditation, using a method of imagination. From this we can infer that any inspiring visualization, religious symbol or form of God pointing to the Self may be part of a practice of Yoga.

We are being asked to concentrate our attention on a reality we haven't learned yet (that there is a Divine Light within). It even requires a certain amount of confidence to seek this out. The visualized Light would gradually disappear and be replaced with the true experience.

37. vitaragavishayan va chittam

Or by reflecting on the mind of a great soul that is fully liberated from connection to objects of sensation.

This can be considered an alternative to the sutra described above. If you can't imagine or believe in your own Inner Light, then look to the heart of a great saint, prophet, or yogi you believe in. Maybe you can see the Light in there.

38. svapnanidrajnanalambanan va

Or had it during dream or deep sleep by concentrating on an insight.

This sutra applies to a particular type of dream: those who are spiritually uplifting, who affect us for the better in some way or who teach us a helpful lesson.

39. yathabhimatadhyanad va

Or by meditating on anything that is uplifting

"As long as you believe it to be spiritually fulfilling, go forward. It is going to work."

40. paramanu paramamahattvantosya vashikarah

Gradually one's concentration mastery extends from the tiniest particle to the greatest magnitude.

The yogi can focus the mind on any aspect of life through faithful practice, from the most subtle to the almost extremely enormous. A mind with that degree of concentration and clarity is suited for infinite meditation.

The next sutra starts a series of four on the subject of samadhi.

41.ksheennavritterabhijatasyevmanergrahitrigrahannagrayeshutatsthatadangjanatasamapattih

Just as the naturally pure crystal assumes the shapes and colors of objects placed near it, so is the mind of the yogi, with its totally weakened modifications, becomes clear and balanced and reaches the state without distinguishing between different forms of knowledge,. That meditation culmination is samadhi.

Why would we want to enter a "world without intelligence, knowledge, and knowledge differentiation?"

As stated in the Sutra 1.17 meaning, perception involves three factors: the knower; an entity to be perceived; and the act of awareness. This triple process is useful to obtain ordinary knowledge, but it is insufficient to experience Prakriti's subtle aspects and to achieve self-realization.

Samadhi is the zenith of the meditative cycle in which the "knower, knowable, and awareness distinction" dissolves. It is a state in which insight is gained through union with the contemplative object. The subconscious, calm and simple as a crystal, momentarily surrenders its self-identity and seems to vanish as it allows the focus of contemplation to shine out alone.

42. tatra shabdarthajnanavikalpaih sankeerna savitarka samapattih

The samadhi in which an object is mixed, its name, and conceptual knowledge of it is called savitarka samadhi, the samadhi with exam.

Savitarka samadhi is absorption on a gross object; one which the ordinary senses can perceive. That absorption initiates a spontaneous and intuitive examination of the contemplated object's qualities. There is union with the object of contemplation, but the word used to designate the object is mixed or interspersed with our learned knowledge of that object.

Savitarka samadhi also offers an intuitive understanding of the sense-perception phenomena. Everything we perceive as the basic perception of any entity is a mixture of three distinct components: name, form, and knowledge:

- Name (sabda): the "hook" we use to grasp outside items

- Entity (artha): the original subject of perception as it exists

- Knowledge (jnana): the chitta's reaction to the object. Knowledge acquired in the ordinary way is the result of the senses that relay an object's vibrations into the mind-stuff, which react by forming vrittis. What we perceive in the mind is not the outside object but the risen modifications. Moreover, past impressions concerning that object pop up. In the chitta, the total sum of this reaction is conceptual knowledge. Conceptual knowledge can be a mixture of precise and erroneous ideas concerning the object being examined. The triple process usually happens so quickly that the measures blend into what seems to be the single event that we call experience

43..smritiparishuddhau.svaroopashoonyevarthamatranirbhasa nirvitarka

When the subconscious is removed from memories (with respect to the object of contemplation), the mind seems to lose its own identity, and the object shines out alone. This is samadhi nirvitarka, the samadhi beyond test.

This is the second of the two samadhis Tarka. The prefix, nir, means "without," but in the context of the Yoga Sutras, it may be best understood as "beyond." As with savitarka samadhi, the object of contemplation is an object perceptible by the senses. Nirvitarka samadhi differs in the sense that the object is now fully known, so the process of "examination" is complete and hence comes to a halt.

In nirvitarka samadhi, the name of the object and any perceptual knowledge of it that was filtered (and therefore skewed or limited) through ordinary thought processes cease to be influential factors in cognition. We are left with just the object as it exists, uncol-ored by any past impressions we have of it. The subjective experience of nirvitarka samadhi is that the mind gives up its own identity for the sake of union of the individual with the object of contemplation.

44. etayaiva savichara nirvichara cha sookshmavishaya vyakhyata

In the same way, savichara (with insight) and nirvichara (beyond insight) samadhis, which are practiced upon subtle objects, are explained. The two chara samadhis parallel the tarka samadhis except that the objects of contemplation are subtle elements (tanmatras), such as the energies or potentials that make sound, touch, taste, color, and sight possible, rather than objects perceivable by the senses. Specifically, savichara samadhi begins the process of understanding the causes that brought the object into being: the subtle elements and the factors of space and time. Nirvichara samadhi is said to be "beyond insight," meaning that there are no further insights into the nature of the object to be had. There is complete knowledge of the object of contemplation down to its subtle essence.

45. sookshmavishayatvan chalinggaparyavasanam

The subtlety of possible objects of concentration ends only at the undifferentiated. The mind gains the ability to focus and merge with every object in creation, down to undifferentiated Prakriti.

46. ta eva sabijah samadhih

All these samadhis are sabija [with seed]. The "seeds" are the subconscious impressions remaining in the mind. They can sprout at any time, given the proper time, place, circumstance, and karma. When they do sprout, they can deprive the mind of the intuitive knowledge of samadhi and reopen the door to the influence of ignorance and egoism.

47 nirvicharavaisharadye adhyatmaprasadah

In the pure clarity of nirvichara samadhi, the supreme Self shines. Although not conferring liberation, nirvichara samadhi, by virtue of its purifying action on the subconscious mind, allows the Self to reflect undistorted on the mind. A unique and subtle wisdom emerges from nirvichara samadhi…

48. rtanbhara tatr prajna

This is ritambhara prajna [the truth-bearing wisdom]. Ritambhara prajna: ritam, "truth," bhara, "bearing," and prajna, "wisdom, knowledge," hence ritambhara prajna, the intuitive wisdom that is truth-bearing.

49..shrutanumanaprajnabhyam.anyavishayaa vishesharthatvat

The purpose of this special wisdom is different from the insights gained by study of sacred tradition and inference. Nirvichara samadhi unlocks the door to Self-realization. In this samadhi, the

Self clearly reflects on the mind and confers a truth-bearing wisdom: the discernment of Purusha from Prakriti. This discernment cannot be achieved through study and inference. Its source is the intuitive insight of nirvichara samadhi.

50. tajjah sanskaro nyasanskarapratibandhi

Other impressions are overcome by the impression produced by this samadhi. This samadhi generates powerful subconscious impressions that incline the mind toward uninterrupted stillness, mastery, and ultimately spiritual union. The "other impressions" mentioned in this sutra, the ones that are overcome, are those that maintain the mind's deeply ingrained habit of externally oriented behavior. The reason that nirvichara samadhi has this overpowering impact on lifetimes of latent subconscious impressions is because the impressions it gener-ates are "truth-bearing," supercharged with the reality and immediacy of the Self.

51. tasyapi nirodhe sarvanirodhannirbijah samadhih

With the stilling of even this impression, every impression is wiped out, and there is nirbija [seedless] samadhi. The finite mind cannot grasp the Infinite. The mind needs to be transcended to reach the final stage, nirbija samadhi. Even the impression left by nirvichara samadhi needs to be transcended. With both conscious mental activity and subconscious impressions (samskaras) completely stilled, the mind achieves (more correctly, realizes) perfect union with the Self. The universe and Self melt into the experience of Oneness.

This truth is expressed in the Vedas as: "Brahman [God or the Absolute] is one without a second." That is, all there is, is God. We can't normally think of one single unit of something without comparing it to at least one more. For example, only one apple (the unity or singularity of it) is impossible to understand unless we can equate it to two or more apples. Even in order to understand the notion of nothing, we must equate it to something. Similarly, by using mind, which operates only with dualities and relativities, we cannot understand the unity of the Absolute.

Samadhi Nirbija is the feeling of total harmony with the Absolute. You realize you've never been born and never will die.

CHAPTER TWO
SADHANA PADA

1. tapahsvadhyayeshvarapranidhanani kriyayogah

During practice, accepting pain as a help to purify, study, and surrender to the Supreme Being constitutes Yoga.

The practices listed in this sutra, named Kriya Yoga, are the context in which all other practices of yoga are placed. They are, in general, the cornerstone of spiritual life and function as training for the eight Yoga limbs (see sutra 2.29).

Kriya Yoga's three aspects are a synergistic combination of:

• Tapas: acceptance of challenges as an aid to purification

• Svadhyaya: refinement of the intellect through introspection and the acquisition of knowledge (study)

• Ishwara Pranidhana: leading a life dedicated to God (self-surrender) Acceptance of pain as an aid to purification: tapas, no one wants to suffer, yet the first word is "purification." We are challenged to actively engage life with an outlook that may seem far-fetched: in which anything that happens can be used for spiritual growth — no matter how painful. In a way, though not always readily apparent, it's all truly for the good— our good. Tapa isn't resignation, a passive concession to life's sorrows; rather it's accepting suffering as a friend and teacher.

Only when we realize that pain— psychological or physical — is a sign that we have reached a limitation within ourselves does tapas start to make sense. Stretch out a muscle beyond its tissue limits, and we feel pain. Push the mind to be just and proper beyond the limits of what it perceives, and we experience suffering. But we need to surmount our limitations to be free. They must be revealed, tested, and uprooted (a process, by the way, greatly supported by studying and surrendering to God). While some of our shortcomings are obvious, however, many others remain hidden in the subconscious, where they do their mischievous work. Through pushing them to emerge in the conscious mind, tapas seeks to reveal latent shortcomings. Suffering, taken with the right understanding, will bring about the effort to overcome limitations. It also encourages introspection and imagination. For instance, it can help us find new, meaningful ways to convince and entice us to sit down for daily meditation or to discover a lesson concealed in our chronic illness that will bring us peace of mind.

2. samadhibhavanarthah kleshatanookaranarthashch

They help us eliminate the obstacles and attain samadhi.

Yoga's aim is not to obtain something that is lacking; it is the realization of a reality that is already present. Practice of yoga does not directly bring about samadhi— it removes the obstacles that impede its experience.

Similar Sutra: 1.29: Describes the way of overcoming the obstacles mentioned as "mind-stuff distractions."

3. avidyasmitaragadveshabhiniveshah kleshaah

The five obstacles are ignorance, selfishness, attachment, aversion and clinging to bodily life.

If our true nature is peace and joy, then what else could be the cause of all our suffering but ignorance?

This sutra addresses the subject of obstacles once again (see sutra 1.30), but on a deeper level. Here, the word klesa is used to designate them, meaning affliction, suffering and pain. Affliction is a fitting term for klesas. They are like a genetic disorder that's tormenting us all our lives.

Like the earlier list of barriers, the klesas are a chain reaction: • The process starts with ignorance. Ignorance is the lack of self-consciousness which leads to self-identity (body-ment).

• Ignorance leads to selfishness. The Self now lost in peace and fulfillment, the mind becomes restless.

• The ego begins developing attachments to objects or situations, seeking to bring them pleasure. The subconscious is guilty of looking for pleasure externals.

• Aversion is the brother of attachment: avoiding something we think can cause pain or discomfort.

We cling to life in the body, as it is the medium by which the mind (through the sense organs) experiences the pleasure that we seek.

4..avidya/kshetram/uttareshan.prasuptatanuvichchhinnodaranam

Right now, for the others mentioned after it, ignorance is the field, whether they are dormant, feeble, intercepted or sustained.

Our daily life experience suggests that there is a truckload of causes for suffering, but ultimately they are grounded in just one cause— avidya, "ignorance." All the other klesas are born out of our True Identity's ignorance.

5. *nityashuchisukhatmakhyatiravidya*

Right now, ignorance is about the impermanent, the impure as good, the painful as fun, and the non-self as the self.

Spiritual ignorance is the result of projecting infinite Self attributes on that which is finite in nature.

Wizards use misdirection to fool our senses and surprise us. Misdirection in life comes in forms such as name, fame, romance, beauty, youth and financial security. Those goals are harmless if we remember that they are limited and that they can't bring permanent happiness. If we view them as sources of unshakable pleasure, they become harmful.

We need to be able to recognize his forms in order to rid ourselves of ignorance. We'll be able to identify the symptoms of ignorance with this sutra to help us as they surface in our lives.

6. drigdarshanashaktyorekatmatevasmita

Right now, selfishness is the identification of the power of the

Seer (Purusha) with that of the instrument of seeing.

The firstborn of greed as well as selfishness is a case of mistaken identity. It is the confusion between the instrument of seeing, the chitta (individual consciousness) and the organs of sense, with consciousness itself. Think, as an analogy, what could happen if we, the driver, were identified with the driving instrument, our car; if we really thought we were our car. When the car was new we would think we were young and beautiful. And when it's getting older, becoming a cantankerous unreliable jalopy, we'd imagine we'd become weak then crabby. We don't make that mistake, of course; it's not hard to discern that the car isn't us but an instrument that we use. However, the confusion between the perception instrument and the Seer presents a difficult test, because this misidentification is profoundly hypnotic, persistent and omnipresent.

7. sukhanushayi raagah

Right now, attachment is what comes from association with experiences of pleasure.

In this sutra the "he" is nervous.

Attachments are limitations which always cause ignorance (avidya) to be deepened or maintained. We are cravings which deny our Self's peace and joy by insisting that the source of happiness is outer experiences.

It innocently starts the series of events that lead to attachment: we engage in an activity or receive an object and find pleasure in it.

We try to replicate this action or event as a source of happiness. In reality, we always reason that if a bit of the experience is good, it would be better for more. Having conferred the power to bring happiness on pleasurable experiences, we spend time, energy, and resources looking through them to attain and retain happiness. It takes a long time to realize that this approach really does not cause anything to be permanently satisfying.

8. duhkhanushayi dveshah

Right now, aversion is that which follows painful experiences of identity.

Aversion, in turn, is attachment. It's the effort to avoid objects or things that we perceive — or fear — will make us unhappy.

We remember such events in life as being relatively neutral; they typically fall out of our conscious memory. Other experiences are either pleasurable enough or painful enough to set past impressions prominently in our storehouse. Since our main goal is to be content, we tend to run after the one that feels good and ignore the negative. The two-sided coin of inspiration lies largely behind all of our life choices.

On some level it really doesn't sound like a bad life strategy. Who wants to suffer pain? Who takes pleasure in suffering? It may sound reasonable but this approach to living life poses a few problems.

It overlooks or underestimates principle interest. Just because something feels good means it's not right. It might be detrimental to others or to us— whether now or later.

9. svarasavahi vidushopi tatharoodho bhiniveshah

Clinging to life, flowing by one's own potency (because of past experience), exists even in the wise.

"Clinging to life" conjures up images of hanging by our fingertips on the edge of a cliff or a child clutching to her mother desperately for safety.

Clinging to life, abhinivesah, is the desire for bodily existence to be continuous. Looking at this obstacle let's start by looking at the biological instinct of the body to preserve itself.

Our bodies have built-in protective instincts: broken bones mend, our immune system fights infections, our eyes snap when dust blows their way and our hands instinctively reach out to break a fall. This is the same survival instinct that we see in a flower bending towards sunlight for warmth or a tree whose roots grow in search of moisture around boulders. While it is true that Nature is expending enormous energy to preserve life, instinctual acts of self-preservation taken by themselves do not constitute the "clinging" of which this sutra is spoken. Clinging requires attachment— an emotional dependency induced by:

- Fear of death

- The habit of relying on self-effort to maintain our lives

- Reliance on experiences of meaning for pleasure

- Recollections of dying in the past

10. te pratiprasavaheyah sookshmah

Such barriers can be overcome in their subtle form by transforming them back into their original cause (the ego).

Resolving the obstacles to their original cause refers to the Self-realization experience in which the mind is transcended and ignorance eradicated. Since ignorance gave birth to the obstacles and sustains them, the obstacles may no longer exist when it is dispelled by the light of the Self.

11. dhyanaheyastadvrittayah

We may be killed in active state by meditation.

Obstacles in the active state are referred to as "intercepted" and "sustained" in sutra 2.4: those obstructions which have noticeable presence and impact on the conscious mind. Meditation (dhyana) prevents awareness from the obstacles that will gradually disappear due to lack of attention.

12..kleshamoolah.karmashayo.drishtadrishtajanmavedaniyah

In these obstacles the womb of karmas has its roots, and the karmas bring experiences in the births seen (present) or in the unseen (future).

Karma is the universal law of cause and effect; of action and reaction. There's a connection between acts and experiences.

As a central tenet of Hindu thought, Sri Patanjali's students were possibly as familiar with karma as the concept of sin is for those in a culture dominated by Judeo-Christians. Most likely, they learned that karma is the universal law of cause and effect, and understood that their karma binds them through embroiling them in the world of relative, material existence. Also, the implacable loops of action and reaction would be known as the cause of reincarnation.

The idea, however, that karma is ingrained in the barriers, which in effect are embedded in ignorance— that karma cannot work without ignorance — might have been disturbing or perhaps a revelation. It meant they couldn't blame for their bad luck or suffering an imper-sonal, unmeasurable, cosmic payback system — or anyone else in that respect. They then confronted what we now face: that all experiences of pleasure and pain are and have always been in our own hands (see sutra 2.14, "The karmas bear the fruits of merit and demerit-caused pleasure and pain"). Though this knowledge clarifies karma's "what and how," it does not describe the "why." Karma is the universal rule that encourages learning.

Any encounter with a piece of information is a cause which impacts our lives. Rain falls (cause); seeds sprout (effect); some herbs lower blood pressure; deep, regulated breathing calms the mind; too much cheesecake causes stomach ache; stress causes headache. Knowledge is the result of observing relationships— the impact on one another by objects, circumstances, and actions. Karma is the cosmic mechanism God has instituted for teaching us. Its ultimate purpose is to guide us towards enlightenment.

13. sati moole tadvipako jatyayurbhogah

There will also be fruits with the existence of the root: the births of various life species, their life spans and experiences.

The Root Ignorance gives birth to the egoism, the small "I."

The birth of the individual produces a psychological "big bang." Something has to be the "I." Could be the only reason "I" is here. When it happens here, there are surfaces. This is accompanied by a series of dualities: you, it, up, down, in, out, good, evil, etc. The appearance of the whole universe rests on the existence of "I."

The Fruits: Births of Different Life Species, Life Spans, and Experiences

Our past thoughts, words, and deeds have brought forth who we are now. What we are doing now determines who we are going to be next. Karma decides whether we are male or female, whether we are rich or poor, whether we are brilliant or dull-witted— even if we are in a human form. It also discourages the lengths of our lives as well as the interactions that come to us.

This does not mean we don't have control over what's going on in our lives. All the time our decisions create new karmas. The future is rooted in our present thoughts, words, and deeds and exists as an infinite possibilities universe.

14. te hladaparitapafalah punyapunyahetutvat

The karmas hold the fruits of pleasure and pain that merit and demerit bring.

This sutra builds upon the previous one's last word—experiences. The nature of the experiences that we will have one day: our successes and failures, the obstacles and unexpected blessings that we will encounter, the friends and enemies and how much we may suffer or rejoice are all contained in that simple word.

Meritorious acts bring pleasurable experiences; on the other hand, they bring painful ones with negative acts. Thus what we experience is based on our own past actions— in this lifetime or in a previous one. Meritorious acts include those based on yama and niyama's moral and ethical principles, and the "four locks and four keys" (see sutras 2.29 and 1.33).

The next sutra brings us beyond the normal preoccupations of pleasure and pain.

15. arinamatapasanskaraduhkhairgunnavritti - virodhaccha duhkham eva sarvan vivekinah

Needless to say, everything is also painful to one of oppression, because of its consequences: the distress and fear of losing what is gained; the resulting memories left in the mind to produce revived cravings; and the tension between the gunas ' actions, which dominate the mind.

This sutra describes how frustration, desire and pain work inside. It presents essentially the same message as the first two of the Four Noble Truths of Lord Buddha: in life, suffering is inevitable; and, second, that suffering is caused. (Looking forward, the next sutra is like the third of the Four Noble Truths: there is a way out of that suffering; and in this Pada, sutra 2.26 introduces unjust discernment as a way out of ignorance.)

16. heyan duhkham anagatam

Pain which has not yet come can be avoided.

A word of optimism after what could become a somewhat gloomy sutra. If pain can be avoided it means we can do something to create a better fate for ourselves. The choices we make in life decide what joy or misery we feel.

17. drashtridrishyayoh sanyogo heyahetuh

The union of the Seer (Purusha) and seen (Prakriti) is the source of that avoidable pain.

It might seem paradoxical for Sri Patanjali to quote as the cause of pain "the union of the Seer and viewed." After all, is union — yoga— not what we're looking for? This sutra seems to suggest that Oneness is the cause of suffering, rather than bringing the end of ignorance and pain.

If we replace the word "union" with "confusion," it might be clearer. Samyoga, translated as union, also means "correlation or connection." In this context, it represents the fundamental inappropriate or false correlation: to mistake for the Seer the mind-stuff that is part of Prakriti. If we think we are the mind, we tend to make choices that serve their whims, fears and habits. We search for things of sense— the "seen "— to offer health, joy, and knowledge, to give us what they can't. This misguided approach to life is the cause of pain and is rooted in (avidya) ignorance.

18..prakashakriyasthitishilan.bhootendriyatmakan bhogapavargarthan drishyam

The view is of gunas nature: enlightenment, development, and inertia. It consists of the elements and organs of sense whose function is to provide the Purusha with both experiences and liberation.

The "seen" is Nature or Prakriti ("to make or do" from the verb root, kr, and pra, out," "to bring forth). As the stuff of creation, it is the source of all that becomes for the Self an object of perception.

The phrase ending this sutra offers an answer to a question that has fascinated humanity from time immemorial: What is life's purpose? Our lives are being played out at the universe's material stage. Why would it have to be so? Why were we put in here? Are all the good and bad times, decisions, events, successes and defeats of our lives leading us to an objective? Or is life a random series of events, with our free will trying to build ease, health, chaos and joy?

Each and every case, glorious or hard to bear, is packed with meaning for the yogi. All that happens is for the Purusha's purpose of giving experiences.

19. visheshavisheshalinggamatralinggani gunnaparvani

The guna stages are common, unspecified, described, and undifferentiated.

Sutra 2.17 claimed that the source of our pain is the Seer's and seen uncertainty, suggesting that the difference between the two is not always discernible. To help end our frustration, we'll look at the evolution of Prakriti from unmanifest to manifest in four phases. These four stages are signposts that help us trace back to the Seer's very doorstep our everyday experience of the solid, three-dimensional world in which we live.

20. drashta drishimatrah shuddhopi pratyayanupashyah

The Seer is nothing but the power of seeing that appears to be seeing through the mind, even if pure.

The Seer is the power of seeing, of consciousness itself, of consciousness, of Purusha, of self.

The subconscious does not have its own consciousness. The consciousness is borrowed from the Seer. This can be compared to the reflection of the sun in a mirror. The Sun stands for the Self; the mirror corresponds to the mind. Though unmeasurable in relation to a mirror, the entire globe of the sun may be reflected in it. We can't say properly though that the sun is in the mirror. The sun is not limited by being reflected, nor its nature altered. This remains pure and untouched.

21. tadarth eva drishyasyatma

The seen remains just for the Seer's sake.

Using the language of the devotee, we may claim that the object of creation — why life exists at all — is to fulfill its Creator's intent which we know is the liberation of the person (see sutra 2.18).

There is no simple, satisfactory answer to why life is like this. The answer to this question lies beyond mind's grasp. It is one of many spiritual puzzles, the solutions to which we will discover not through logic but through ignorance transcendent.

22. kritarthan prati nashtam apyanashtan tadanyasadharannatvat

Though destroyed for the one who has attained freedom, for others it (the seen) remains, being familiar to them.

Objects enjoy an existence that is not dependent upon the perception of them by any individual. The tree outside my window exists whether or not I perceive it because the same tree will be experienced by any person walking by my home. So, this sutra does not speak of universe destruction. It describes a change in the relation with the universe of the realized yogi. Until liberation, Prakriti built an infinite storehouse of meaning objects that the mind wanted to bring happiness, and that we mistakenly believed may occur. With the achievement of freedom, Prakriti is losing its central place in life, not having the same importance any more.

23. svasvamishaktyoh svaroopopalabdhihetuh sanyogah

Owner (Purusha) and owned (Prakriti) union causes them both to recognize their nature and powers.

In the phenomenon that we experience as life the Purusha and Prakriti are allies. This partnership forms the basis for knowledge acquisition. The basic consciousness which is the Purusha allows for object awareness to occur. And it's the mind's ability to discern Prakriti's changing nature that leads to gaining knowledge about and realization of the Purusha.

24. tasya heturavidya

Ignorance is the cause of that union.

The Owner's and owned union in the previous sutra sounded like a nice situation, a source of knowledge. And that is on the relative level. But as long as we remain ignorant of our True Identity, however much we learn about the universe and study the nature of the Self, we are subject to suffering.

25. tadabhavat sanyogabhavo hanan taddrisheh kaivalyam

Practices of yoga gradually strip away ignorance. The alliance between Purusha and Prakriti ends with the departure of ignorance, and along with it, the mistaken self-identification for Self. The source of suffering is destroyed and we, jivanmuktas, become free beings. (See sutra 4.34, which goes into more detail on this state).

26. vivekakhyatiraviplava hanopayah

The tool for its elimination is continuous discriminative discernment.

Discriminatory discernment is an inherent skill, viveka. We recognize it in our everyday life as the ability to discern the unique characteristics of an entity, or the difference between two or more objects. Our discriminative capacity is usually occupied with a constant stream of relevant and irrelevant thoughts: perceptions of objects, events, wishes and people flowing into consciousness. But to perceive the Self as our True Identity, to pierce through ignorance, viveka requires a high order of clear, steady focus and the absence of selfish attachment. The more focused our minds become, the more our ability to "see" becomes refined, subtle and complete. As we continue with meditation, prayer, non-attachment and study, we will not only be developing nirodha but also viveka.

Viveka is the transfer of consciousness from an object of perception to the force of perception (Purusha) itself. At the end of the day, it is pure consciousness that knows itself as distinct from any object or experience.

27. tasya saptadhaa prantabhoomih prajna

In the end stage, one's experience is sevenfold.

The viveka practice changes the way we view life. Our perception will reveal a different self and universe than those we previously knew.

What is to be avoided (the causes of suffering) is recognised through the practice of viveka.

28. yogangganushthanad ashuddhikshaye jnanadiptira vivekakhyateh

The impurities dwindle away by the practice of the Yoga limbs and there dawns the light of wisdom which leads to discriminative discernment.

Note the series of occurrences:

• Yoga limb activities eliminate impurities. Yoga activities do not bring something new; they do away with unwanted or needless stuff.

• Wisdom appears as impurities dwindle, meaning that wisdom already resides inside. The light of wisdom (jnanadipti) in this sutra relates to insights into the spiritual truths. As far as the practice of Yoga is concerned, knowledge enables the ability to recognize the target, set our path on the right track and keep it there.

• Wisdom leads to viveka, as we saw in sutra 2.26, which is the method of removing ignorance.

29..yamaniyamasanapranayamapratyaharadharanadhyanasamadhayo-a-shtava anggani

The eight Yoga limbs are:

1. Yama–withdrawal

2. Niyama- Comment.

3. Asana-Position

4. Pranayama-control of breath

5. Pratyahara-withdrawal of meaning

6. Dharan focus.

7. Dhyana–to meditate

8. Samadhi–Contemplation, meditation or superconscious state, eight limbs seamlessly integrate selfless, active involvement in life with introspection and contemplation. This delicate balance is intended to promote self-knowledge, extend and transform

consciousness, and culminate in self-realisation.

30. ahinsasatyasteyabrahmacharyaparigraha yamah

Yama is Nonviolence, Truthfulness, Non-Stealing, Continence and Nongreed.

What attitudes precede enlightened actions? One born of selfless motivations, wisdom, and love, seeking the welcoming will of all involved. These same attitudes— the yamas listed here — are virtues that strengthen and purify the mind.

Yama concepts might not satisfy somebody who likes a dos and don'ts list. We are known more accurately as strategies for actions — attitudes that bring clarity, concentration and objectivity to bear on all circumstances.

We will eventually know them well enough to call them friends if we allow these concepts to direct, cajole and correct us. We'll be deprived of their nature, intent, power, and meaning— their spirit. Only when we interpret the meaning behind the "letter of law" do we truly understand the yamas.

31. jatideshakalasamayanavachchhinnah sarvabhauma mahavratam

These Great Vows are universal and not limited by class, location, time or circumstance.

This sutra underscores the importance of the yamas. They are even accentuated by the niyamas, because they apply to everybody, whether they are spiritual seekers or not. These are guiding principles for anyone irrespective of their occupation, status, location, time of day, year, or life, or the context. They are as valid today as they were thousands of years ago, as they overcome all conditions and challenges.

32. shauchasantoshatapahsvadhyayeshvara-pranidhanani niyamah

Niyama consists of simplicity, contentment, acknowledging but not causing God's (self-surrender) suffering, analysis and adoration.

The word niyama expresses the essential principles governing spiritual growth. While the yamas are universal — for all in all situations and stages of life — the niyamas are especially important practices for spiritual seekers who wish to prepare the mind for self-realisation.

33. vitarkabadhane pratipakshabhavanam

When distracted by negative thoughts, it is necessary to think of opposite (positive) ones. This is bhavana with pratipaksha.

34. vitarkaa hinsadayah kritakaritanumodita lobhakrodhamohapoorvaka mridumadhyadhimatra duhkhajnananantafala iti pratipakshabhavanam

Whether incited by greed, anger, or infatuation, whether indulged in mild, medi-um, or extreme intensity, they are based on ignorance and bring some pain when negative thoughts or acts such as violence and so on are caused to be done or even approved of. Thus reflecting is pratipaksha bhavana, too.

Negative thoughts or actions apply to those who condemn the yamas and niyamas. Yoga provides two invaluable methods for reducing negativity: a cure to be taken while in the midst of depressive events and a safeguard that immunizes the mind from its recurrence.

35. ahimsapratishthayam tatsannidhau vairatyagah

All hostilities end in the presence of one which is firmly established in nonviolence.

The mindful fight to overcome gross and subtle tendencies of aggression is an advanced study of the psychology of violence. Yogis experience for themselves through these personal struggles that fear breeds anger and that anger ruins our peace and clarity. Yogis therefore understand the pain that violence brings and know this pain is something that we all share. Their empathy for others' suffering brings compassion, naturally. With the passing of time, compassion gives birth to such pure love and understanding that it raises the mind to a place of peace beyond any tranquility we had imagined. The powerful healing energy of love and understanding then flows from an area of greater to lesser concentration in a process similar to osmosis. The calming influence of selfless love is a powerful and palpable natural emanation which flows into the hearts of others from the hearts of those who are perfected in nonviolence. It is in their presence that fear and discord vanish.

36. satyapratishthayam kriyafalashrayatvam

The acts and their effects are subordinate to one defined in truthfulness.

The yogi attain harmony with reality. There can be no doubt that anything not supposed to be said. Whatever the fact is she says. Each whisper of the Divine Will quickly shifts her mind, like feathers blown by the wind.

37. asteyapratishthayam sarvaratnopasthanam

To one that doesn't steal, all wealth comes.

Aside from keeping our hands out of unauthorized cookie jars, no stealing perfection includes not improperly benefiting from the thoughts or ideas of another. No stealing brings about a transition from constant desire for more to contentment with what is offered to us and eventually kindness. Generosity is what leads to the richness that this sutra mentioned. The more selflessly we donate, the more we get. It is karma practice, and also good business.

38. brahmacharyapratishthayam viryalabhah

Vigor is gained towards one's establishment in continence.

We gain vigour when we don't waste energy. It's not just that we're going to have more energy but it's going to be more subtle, stable and healing quality. It is the sort of energy that others will feel in our presence, radiating naturally like light or heat.

39. aparigrahasthairye janmakathantasanbodhah

A detailed illumination of the how and why of one's birth comes to one deeply rooted in non-greed.

We gain the ability to see how our impulses influence what we do in life when we are free of greed. Not only will we discover how previous cravings brought certain experiences in this birth, but how powerful past desires propelled us into this one from our past life.

40. shauchat svanggajugupsa parairasansargah

The defensive instincts of the body are activated by purification, as well as disinclination to the adverse interaction with others.

This is the first of two sutras describing the advantages of pureness.

There is some confusion surrounding this sutra, especially with regard to the meaning of the phrase, jugupsa, usually translated as "disgust." Let's look at a word-for-word translation: Sauchat, "purification" Svanga, "one's own body" Jugupsa, "that which inspires defense," derived from, ju, "to urge, encourage, continue," gup, "to guard, defend, preserve," and sa= "procure, confer" We would immediately spit out, for example, a mouthful of crude oil. Don't confuse disgust with personal preference. A dislike of red cabbage is not an abomination. No matter how objectionable it may be to our taste buds, it's a matter of personal preference to reject red cabbage for dinner.

41. sattvashuddhisaumanasyaikagryendriyajayatmadars hanayojnatvani cha

In addition, one achieves sattwa integrity, mind cheerfulness, one-pointing, sensory awareness, and self-realization health.

The list of mental purity benefits given in this sutra contains two elements that are reminiscent of the two-pronged approach described in sutra 1.12 for achieving nirodha: practice and nonattachment. In this sutra we hear that purity fosters one-point mind (see sutra 1.13) and sensual mastery (see sutras 1.15 and 1.16).

42. santoshad anuttamah sukhalabhah

Supreme happiness is achieved through contentment.

In the lack of cravings, contentment is mastered. It is the belief that nothing is lost, that all that happens is part and parcel of a Divine Plan. The consequence is happiness transcending transitory pleasures and almost exactly representing the Self's absolute bliss.

Happiness is not a gift or an event mistakenly bestowed by a capricious God. It is the product of cultivating a vision of life which "sees" the unity of the Self behind the different names and forms.

43. kayendriyasiddhirashuddhikshayat tapasah

Body and sensual impurities are eliminated by austerity, and supernatural powers are acquired.

Austerity is the struggle to live by the values that we have set before us, and to embrace whatever life brings our way. It is a process which is strengthening and purifying us.

In addition to physical toxins, impurities include the obstacles of sutra 1.30, anything which opposes the spirit of the yamas and niyamas (sutras 2.30 and 2.32), and the source of all impurities, ignorance of the Self (sutras 2.3 and 2.4, the klesas).

44. svadhyayad ishtadevatasanprayogah

Communion with one's chosen deity comes through study.

In this sutra, there are three important ideas to consider: Deity, Selected, and Communion.

Deity

The Sutras of Yoga do not advocate any particular form of God to worry because the yogi understands every deity as Ishwara's manifestation and worthy of veneration. Thus, every God name and form can be a gateway to higher spiritual experiences.

Chosen

The deity chosen, ishta devata, is common feature of Hinduism. Seekers are free to choose whatever name and form appeals to them as objects of their devotion.

It is understood that certain qualities are prominently associated with a particular deity which may resonate deep within the devotee. The right to worship God in whatever form we want provides the benefit of being able to establish a romantic relationship-ship with the Divine more easily. There will also be our energy, our thinking and our actions where the heart is. Loving never goes idle. It begets sadhana in this case, and communion with the Absolute.

Communion

The receptiveness and focus acquired by research consumes the mind in any dimension of the Absolute with which the seeker has built a devoted relationship. This experience can also be the product of repetition of a mantra linked to the focus of devotion of the seeker.

Communion with one's chosen deity also suggests imbibing the deity's associated qualities.

45. samadhisiddhirishvarapranidhanat

Samadhi is attained by total surrendering to Ishwara.

One day, every spiritual path brings us face to face with the unadulterated ego. We view it in all its obstinate glory. But if we want to realize the Infinite Self as our True Identity, we have to transcend the ego-limit. The problem is that efforts to transcend the ego often cause it to emphatically reassert itself as the fear that if we proceed, we will cease to exist.

Surrendering to Ishwara is the easiest way to overcome this obstacle, because it is not based on having the power of will to overcome the threat of annihilation to transcend the ego. Instead, the ego is absorbed in loving reverence and moves readily towards union with the beloved Divine.

Similar Sutra: 1.23: It describes Ishwara's first time surrender as a way to achieve samadhi.

46. sthirasukham aasanam

Asana is a relaxed, steady pose.

It applies to formally seated postures in meditation and implies that we should find or maintain a position that leaves us free to focus the mind and breathe without the intrusion of aches, pains or restlessness.

Hatha Yoga's bending and relaxing postures are effective ways to achieve "asana."

47. prayatnashaithilyanantasamapattibhyam

Through minimizing the natural tendency to restlessness, and meditating on the infinite, posture is mastered. We feel a gradual lessening of restlessness when we sit in a relaxed, steady asana and concentrate on the Infinite. This happens when we concentrate on something that is immovable and whose limits for us are unmeasurable

This sutra has a symbolic meaning, too. Ananta (the word translated as "infinite") is also the name of the cosmic snake which symbolizes Lord Vishnu's strength. Lord Vishnu is often depicted as being seated on Ananta, whose various hooded heads spread open to form a canopy over the head of the Lord. The waters of life are all around Lord Vishnu— a churning, spinning, restless ocean. Lord Vishnu is the Creator, and Ananta represents the universe's strength at His feet and His pleasure. Such symbols indicate that we gain Divine Power (symbolized by Lord Vishnu) when we put under our control the natural tendency to restlessness (the churning ocean of energy or prana) by meditating and tapping into the infinite source of inner power (represented by Ananta).

48. tato dvandvanabhighatah

Thereafter, one is undisturbed by dualities.

To enter the Self's deeper truth, the mind needs to be free from dualities— heat and cold, up and down, in and out, and so forth. This is an essential prerequisite for pranayama's subtler perceptions, detachment of the mind, and contemplation.

This sutra indicates the object of asana practice is not merely a physical but also a mental one.

49. tasmin sati shvasaprashvasayorgativichchhedah pranayamah

The movements of inhalation and exhalation should be monitored for that (firm posture) being acquired. This is pranayama.

Pranayama, by air, is mastery of prana, the universal life force. Breath movements reflect prana status in the body-mind. Irregular respiration is suggestive of imbalances or block-age in prana flow. The prana flows in the appropriate measure and locations by regulation of the breath. Blockages are removed, the energy is increased and health improved.

In sutra 2.15, we discovered that it is difficult to be permanently satisfied unless the gunas are controlled: "To one of injustice, yes, everything is painful because of its effects... the constant conflict between the gunas ' actions, which dominate the mind." Pranayama is of vital importance to this effort because it helps to bring the gunas into a balanced state.

50. bahyabhyantarastambhavrittih deshakalasankhyabhih paridrishto dirghasookshmah

Life-breathing modifications are external, internal, or stationary. We are to be regulated by space, time, and number and are long or short.

In general, in relation to the body, our breath rotates between three different movements: towards it, away from it, and fixed (the mechanisms of breathing become still).

Space refers to the mental focal point during the practice. The prana flows wherever attention goes. The attention is either directed to areas such as the base of the spine or between the eye-brows, or maybe where the practitioner feels there is a lack of prana when healing is intended.

Time means the length of time the breath is inhaled, exhaled, and held.

Number refers to the number of individual practice reps and rounds.

The three breath-taking modifications — inhalation, exhalation, and retention— can be controlled and governed to promote improvement in pranayama practice.

51. bahyabhyantaravishayakshepi chaturthah

There is a fourth kind of pranayama that occurs on an internal or external body during con-centration. It is referred to as a natural, effortless state of breath suspension that occurs during deep meditation, called kevala kumbhaka. Since the breath represents the state of the body and mind, the breath usually stops for a while when the body becomes fully still and comfortable and the mind is quiet and clear.

52. tatah ksiyate prakasa varanam

As a consequence, the veil is broken over the inner light.

Prakasa, translated as interior light, refers to the sattwa guna standard. As tamas, or darkness, disperses it shines out.

All our thoughts can be categorized according to the gunas ' qualities— tamas, rajas, and sattwa. Thoughts characterized by sluggishness, carelessness, or lack of attention are tamasic and characterized as heavy and restraining movement. Rajasic thoughts are agitated, and by erratic focus and powerful emotions mask the Self. The pranayama practice helps counteract tamas inertia and rajas restlessness. Sattwa predominates as rajas and tamas decay. Although the veils that cover the Self are now more transparent, the fullness of the Self is still hidden by sattwa's engaging but transitory gladness.

53. dharanasu ca yogyata manasah

And the mind becomes fit for focus.

More sattwa means more medita-tion peace, clarity and steadiness. Through reality the mind finds joy because it encounters some nice thing. It's becoming easier to focus your mind.

54. svasvavishayasanprayoge chittasy svaroopanukarivendriyanan pratyaharah

This is pratyahara, when the senses detach from the objects and mimic, as it were, the essence of the mind-stuff.

The senses do not function independently of the mind; thus, they detach from their objects when the focus is drawn inward and also go inward.

The senses are openings through which the mind-stuff enters information. But perception only occurs when the mind "joins" with the senses. No perception can happen without the union of mind and senses. For example, when the mind is absorbed in a thrilling novel we don't notice sounds outside of our living room. The sound vibrations still reach the ears, but they do not make any conscious impression on the individual awareness since the mind is engaged elsewhere.

55. tatah parama vasyate ndriyanam

Then, supreme mastery over the senses follows.

As a tortoise pulls in its limbs, the practitioner can withdraw the senses at will. Temptations and cravings are dealt with not by eliminating them, but by turning focus to a better place and keeping it steady.

It is necessary to comprehend that sense-mastery is not a deprivation activity. It is instead the path to greater joy:

CHAPTER THREE
VIBHUTI PADA

1. deshabandhashchittasya dharana

Dharana is the mind binding to one location, one entity or one concept.

In dharana (concentration), the mind turns its focus to a fixed point: some position, entity, or idea chosen by the practitioner. The mind, of course, is not in the habit of focusing attention on one level. It wants to run around here and there, and it does. Often during a session of meditation the subconscious will slither away silently, initially undetected. Each time the wandering ways of the mind are discovered, the practitioner allows the wayward thoughts to go away and refocuses on the meditation object. The mind wanders less often over time and becomes ever quieter, simpler, and stronger.

To let go of intrusive emotions is a characteristic of many practices in Yoga. This technique, for example, is similar to the redirection approach used in pratipaksha bhavana, pratyahara and the form of the four locks and four keys. Regularity in these practices will therefore serve as an aid to advancement in dharana.

2. tatra pratyayaikatanata dhyanam

Dhyana is the continuous cognitive flow toward that object.

As dharana is continuous it eventually becomes dhyana, the

proper meditation state, immediately. No other thoughts intrude during the time that the mind is in the meditative state. At this stage, the mind's web-weaving vritti activity winds down to a halt, and the mind's natural penetrating quality becomes more visible. The process of communion with the object of meditation commences in earnest with dhyana.

It is noteworthy that while attaining dhyana requires effort, when there is no further struggle in that state. Meditation is the natural, easy and unbreakable flow of attention towards the object chosen. The meditative mind is tranquil, clear and focused.

In fact, it is only when the mind has attained all three criteria at the same time that we can say there is meditation status.

3. tad evarthamatranirbhasan svaroopashoonyam iva samadhih

Samadhi is the same meditation when the mind-stuff reflects the object alone, as if it is devoid of its own form.

If the purpose of meditation practice is to acquire knowledge of the immediate, unbiased, and whole object of meditation, then the mind must reach a state where it completely, even if temporarily, surrenders whatever form it holds in favor of that of the object chosen. Having abandoned all resistance to union with the object of contemplation, the mind completely and accurately represents the object's shape in the same way that an undistorted and perfectly clean mirror retains our face's absolute and exact reflection.

The samadhi presented in this sutra does not describe the highest samadhi, nirbija samadhi, which also wipes out all latent subconscious impressions.

4. trayam ekatra sanyamah

The practice of these three (dharana, dhyana, and samadhi) is called samyama upon one object.

Samyama means being controlled to perfection.

Union with the object of meditation occurs when, through successive progression from dharana to dhyana and finally to samadhi, the mind penetrates through. Through samyama, the mind deeply dives into any concept or thought. It gains complete knowledge of the object of interest in the process, down to its subtlest aspects.

5. tajjayat prajnaalokah

Knowledge born from intuition shines forth by the mastery of samyama.

Prajnalokah is the term for "shines out" This consists of prajna, "intuitive understanding or wisdom," and alokah, "brilliance, light." Samyama's learned knowledge is clear and intuitive. It is a bursting forth of the light of the object of meditation— the reality or essential nature. The creation, evolution, and dissolution of any entity is fully revealed.

Samyama is a skill which helps to make a practitioner fit for the transcendent self-knowledge.

6. tasya bhoomishu viniyogah

It accomplishes its practice in stages.

Knowing that there are several stages of achievement, we can assume there are different signposts to help guide and reassure us on the path. These are addressed in sutras 3.9—3.12.

This sutra may also be a gentle admonition addressed to students who, upon hearing of the incredible benefits of samyama practice, think they could begin their practice at this level. Everybody needs to start from the basics. At the same time, it encourages those who feel the samyama practice is too difficult to accomplish by reminding them that the longest journey starts with a single step.

7. trayam antaranggan poorvebhyah

These three (dharana, dhyana, and samadhi) are more internal than the five limbs previous to them.

You need the outside world to practice the yamas and niyamas. You need the body to practice asana and pranayama, which is composed of the gross elements. Pratyahara has only meaning in relation to a world outside of the senses. But in order to practice these last three limbs, the practitioner must go inside and start working with and exploring consciousness itself. Therefore these limbs are considered to be more internal.

8. tad api bahiranggan nirbijasy

Even the seedless samadhi is external to these three.

Until the samadhi nirbija, subconscious experiences remain as seeds which can trigger the effect of ignorance on mental function. Through nirbija samadhi the whole of individual consciousness is still and pure, including the subconscious.

All other samadhis compared with nirbija samadhi are local

9. vyutthananirodhasanskarayorabhibhava-pradurbhavau nirodhakshannachittanvayo nirodhaparinamah

The outward sensations are diluted by the presence of nirodha impressions. As the mind begins to be imbued with moments of nirodha, development is taking place in nirodha.

Like the sunrise which always overpowers night's darkness, nirodha unfailingly counteracts vyutthana, outsourcing. Our efforts are like strong seeds that all contribute in helping to get the job done. No effort is ever wasted in Yoga. Our practices are planting and nourishing seeds of nirodha, quietness and clarity. They sprout, grow and blossom in time.

It is evident that Nirodha performs activities such as meditation, prayer, reading, and self-analysis. But when we establish the inner atmosphere in which nirodha thrives, nirodha really gains momentum. In practice, this means looking at sacred wisdom principles as the standard by which we make choices and by which we adjust our perception of life and of the world.

10. tasya prashantavahita sanskarat

The mind-stuff gets a calm flow of nirodha when impressions of nirodha get strong and pervasive.

It describes a mind in nirodha that has attained effortlessness by routine, devoted effort. No more strain, no more coercing of the mind. A strong subconscious momentum was built toward Self-realization. Such a mind considers it easy to pursue fulfilment inside, to be calmer, more concentrated, and more selfless. The doors to knowledge start to open and confidence eventually grows.

Related Sutra: 1.14: Describes how it creates habits.

11 sarvarthataikagratayoh kshayodayau chittasya samadhiparinamah

As distractions dwindle and focus emerges, the mind-stuff turns toward samadhi.

As time is repeated and prolonged in nirodha, the mind-stuff starts to lose the habit of shifting attention from object to object. It is said to achieve ekagrata, one-pointedness. In samadhi, samadhi parinama, one-pointness marks the beginning of creation.

Samadhi brings significant mental-environmental changes. It's almost like having a house renovated, adding a new floor, more rooms, windows and closets. We see fresh views through new openings, and suddenly find storage spots for all. Our newly renovated house impacts on many functional and emotional aspects in our lives. Similarly, the mind undergoing the samadhi process of transformation begins operating in a state of increased receptivity that opens it to subtle influences, knowledge, and experiences.

12. tatah punah shantoditau tulyapratyayau chittasyaikagrataparinamah

It is important to emphasize that there is focus (ekagrata parinama) when the images that subside and those that arise are identical.

Thought waves still arise, though in a unique way, even if the mind has attained focus. There is a continuous flow of consciousness towards the object of attention where waves of awareness that subside and emerge are similar. It is like watching a fruit bowl when neither the bowl nor the camera is being pushed. Every frame from the last is indisclaimable. In essence, the result would be the same as a still photograph.

It takes the form of the object of meditation when the mind reaches a focused state.

13. etena bhootendriyeshu dharmalakshanavastha parinama vyakhyatah

The transformations of the form, characteristics, and condition of the elements and sense organs are explained by what has been said (in sutras 3.9–3.12).

This sutra focuses on the evolutionary consequences of both time and climate. It gives us a glimpse of the three great tracks along which Nature objects — including the mind— change.

14. shantoditavyapadeshyadharmanupati dharmi

The substratum (Prakriti) remains in existence although it goes through latent, uprising, and unmanifested phases by nature.

Prakriti remains a permanent constant. It is the substratum of all the changes and phases through which objects traverse. Latent (santa or quieted) refers to the object's form(s) now in the past, uprising indicates the present phase, and unmanifested refers to the potential of an object, the transformations that are yet to come.

15. kramanyatvan parinamanyatve hetuh

The succession of these various phases is the cause of the differences in evolutionary stages.

The effects of time and weather on an object, which arise in an organized and predictable way, are the reasons that we see changes (what we call evolution) in natural objects.

The reason we see changes in objects is because the gunas interplay brings changes in the perceivable form of objects; characteristics that have existed in the past (latent) appear in the present (uprising) and wait to be expressed (unmanifested) in the future.

16. parinamatrayasanyamadatitanagatajnanam

Knowledge of past and future comes from practice of samyama on the three stages of evolution.

The yogi can clearly perceive the origin and evolutionary course of any entity or event by focusing on the inner workings of evolution (the conception, creation, and subsidizing of objects in Nature).

Until proceeding with the list of achievements, let's pause to discuss why so many sutras revolve around this samyama activity.

All questions stem directly or indirectly from one: Who am I? This one question gives birth to countless others, like: What is life's nature and the cosmos? When did it commence? What time is it? What is the end of life? All we study, observe and investigate can reveal somewhat about our nature and purpose.

Today, to reveal the mysteries of the universe, we look at scientific methodologies, high-tech instruments, computer analysis, and double-blind trials. Scientific research may have lacked the advantages of advanced instrumentation in the day of Sri Patanjali but exquisitely nuanced observations were made in a different way. The source of matter and the boundaries of the universe have been plumbed to a remarkable degree by harnessing the power of mind.

17. shabdarthapratyayanam itaretaradhyasat sankarah tatpravibhagasanyamat sarvabhootarutajnanam

A term, its context, and the concept behind it are generally confused due to being superimposed on each other. Knowledge of its significance is obtained by samyama on the word (or sound) produced by any being.

We can ascertain the meaning behind any samyama sound or word. What a great Communication Boon! We are privy to any speaker's true motivation. We could understand the intention behind the sounds our pets make, too.

18 sanskarasakshatkaranat poorvajatijnanam

Knowledge of past births is obtained by direct perception, through samyama, of one's mental impressions.

Reincarnation is not just a philosophy or theory that is believed to be comforting, because it makes sense. It is a reality that can be perceived directly (see sutra 1.7, in which direct perception is given as a source of right knowledge).

By turning our attention inward, observing subconscious impressions directly, and noting when, how, and why they are manifesting, we'll see themes, keynote thoughts— the essential plotline around which our current life was formed. If we perceive these themes directly through samyama, we will find that they originated from past actions and latent impressions of past births. By going even further down this path, we will discover that those past impressions were the product of former incarnations.

19. pratyayasy parachittajnanam

Knowledge of their mental images is obtained through samyama on the distinguishing signs of other's bodies.

We have an instinctive reaction (partly due to biological impulses) to other people's physical appearance and form conscious or subconscious impressions about at least certain aspects of their character. For example, we may be wary of people whose eyes are too close together or instinctively know that a fearful type is the person whose shoulders are usually hunched around their ears.

The fact that the appearance of people can be so different when they sleep (when the conscious mind loses its control to the subconscious) suggests that the mental material helps to organize their face's physical structures. In other words, the individual's character determines facial expressions, and the language of the body.

20. na cha tat salambanan,tasyavishayibhootatvat

But this does not include the support in the mind of the person (such as the motive behind the thought, and so on), since that is not the samyama's object.

We may know the nature of the mind from studying the body but not the underlying motivations.

21.kayaroopasanyamat.tadgrahyashaktistambhe.chakshuhprakashasanprayogentardhanam

The body becomes invisible by samyama on the form of one's body (and by) checking the power of perception through interception of light from the observer's eyes.

The ancient yogis understood that waves of light need to be taken in by the senses and passed on to the appropriate brain center in order for perception to take place. In order to perceive it, the eyes must capture the light reflected off an object. Yogis have the ability to intercept the light that reflects off their bodies, making it appear like they have vanished.

22. etena shabdadyantardhanamuktam

The disappearance of sound (and touch, taste, smell, and so on) is clarified in the same way.

It has already been suggested that the Yogi's mastery extends to such subtle areas.

Related Sutra: 1.40: "Gradually one's concentration mastery extends from the tiniest particle to the greatest magnitude."

23. sopakraman nirupakraman cha karma tatsanyamad aparantajnanam, arishtebhyo va

Karmas are of two kinds: to manifest quickly and to manifest slowly. The knowledge of the time of death is obtained by samyama on them, or on the portents of death.

The yogi will perform samyama on the karmic seeds of the subconscious waiting to sprout. Some are suited to this current circumstance of life and quickly come to fruition; others find their growth inconducive to the current life.

Through samyama, yogis directly perceive the karmas that created the present life, and were the basis for vital lessons. Upon completion of the lessons, the yogis know that it is time to graduate from the current birth. They may take another birth in the future after graduating from this birth, or if they have achieved Self-realization, they may simply enjoy their unity with the Absolute.

Knowledge of the time of death can be helpful, as our last thoughts have a strong effect on the essence of possible births. Spiritual thoughts can help to bring forth a birth conducive to spiritual growth, hankering for material success will bring forth a physically comfortable birth, and negative thoughts, an unwanted rebirth.

24. maitryadishu balani

The power to transmit them is obtained by samyama on friendliness, and other such qualities.

This sutra offers a great way to improve one's own life and the lives of others. We can attain its benefits by performing samyama on a desirable quality, like friendliness.

Spiritual history is full of stories of sages and saints whose mere presence has mysteriously changed other people's lives. They often transmitted these virtuous qualities without intention or effort, just as the sun automatically radiates warmth and light, without intention.

This is referred to by the four locks and four keys of sutra 1.33. By implication, we can understand this sutra to mean that we with any virtue can obtain such power.

25. baleshu hastibaladini

Their strength is obtained by samyama on the strength of the elephants and other such animals.

Using a picture like an elephant only helps. One could replace any image that relays the idea of great strength. The underlying principle is that the universe's limitless capacity is accessible to the concentrated mind to tap through.

26. pravrittyalokanyasat sookshmavyavahita-viprakrishtajnanam

Knowledge of the subtle, hidden, and remote is obtained through samyama on the light within. Note: subtle as atoms, hidden as treasure, distant as far-off lands. This samyama's object is not the Self but the light of the Self reflecting on the mind. The inner senses are illuminated by virtue of this samyama, which results in the ability to gain knowledge of things that are present but normally not perceptible.

27. bhuvanajnanan soorye sanyamat

Knowledge of the entire solar system is obtained through samyama on the Sun.

The sun is the center of the solar system, and others depend on it for all life. Know the source and you'll be aware of the manifestations. You can know the whole, by knowing a part; the whole is reflected in the part. This concept is central to Eastern healing modalities, where the practitioner can assess all organs and systems, for example, by taking the pulse, observing the tongue, or palpating the abdomen. Acupuncturists use points on the ear and scalp to treat any part of the body, iridologists may measure all body systems by inspecting the eyes and reflexologists treat imbalances in any part of the body by massaging reflexes on the hands or feet.

28. chandre taravyoohajnanam

Knowledge of the alignment of stars comes from samyama on

the moon.

The alignment of the stars refers to the Constellations.

29. dhruve tadgatijnanam

Knowledge of the movements of the stars comes from samyama on the pole star.

The pole star is fixed in the sky; the stars' movements in relation to it are known. Since we are considering the samyama items and not just ordinary observation or research, the information that Sri Patanjali is talking about gives a definition not only of what is, but of why. In this case the yogi may glimpse the reasons for the stars.

30. nabhichakre kayavyoohajnanam

Knowledge of body constitution is obtained through samyama on the navel plexus.

The navel is the source point we develop from within the womb. Oriental medicine teaches us how to continue recreating from the navel after birth at the energetic level. A detailed system for assessing the health of the body's organs and systems by means of visual and palpatory examination of the abdomen evolved from this knowledge.

31. kanthakoope kshutpipasanivrittih

The cessation of hunger and thirst is achieved through samyama at the throat pit.

This would be a very practical technique for yogis living in caves, forests, or other remote areas and who frequently relied on alms to sustain them.

Some powers, like this one, are not deemed too hard to achieve. They might also serve as tests for practitioners wondering how far their mental mastery has gone.

32. koormanadyan sthairyam

In the meditative motionless posture, it is achieved by samyama on the kurma nadi.

The nadis are prana flows, or vital energy, similar to the Acupuncture meridians. Nadis for the body-mind is a method of contact and control. Kurma nadi, literally, "tortoise-shaped tube," is located underneath the throat and refers to the prana function that closes the eyes. This may symbolize the ability to draw attention away from the outside world

The picture of a tortoise in this sutra indicates that symbolism can be at play.

A tortoise is capable of removing its head and limbs into a protective shell just as a yogi is capable of extracting the senses from daily worries, enabling the mind to become still and calm, and preparing it for meditation.

In India's mythology, the world was said to be supported as it swam through the universe on the back of a cosmic tortoise. It would be known that tortoise represents a solid, steady base.

There is a story about Lord Vishnu, who incarnated as a tortoise to support Mount Mandara, which the heavenly beings needed to stir up the ocean of life to recover the nectar of immortality

33. moordhajyotishi siddhadarshanam

Visions of masters and adepts are obtained by samyama on the light at the head's crown (sahasrara chakra)

When the consciousness is lifted to the crown chakra, it will experience visions of the great saints and sages. Another interpretation is that we obtain the same spiritual vision as the masters when the consciousness functions from the crown chakra. It was not Sri Patanjali who left us with detailed descriptions of these experiences. We are subtle and best left to observe rather than to argue and evaluate.

There are seven major chakras (literally, "wheels"), which are subtle centers of consciousness that are located along the spine from the tailbone to the top of the head although not part of the gross anatomy. We reflect evolutionary levels:

- The chakra at the base of the spine is about self-preservation, our primary instinct as living beings.

- The next chakra, located behind the genitals, relates primarily to reproduction. The desire to procreate arises, once we feel safe.

- In the navel is the chakra which governs will assertion and our interactions with others.

- The 4th chakra is the heart, the center of compassion. It is the middle chakra, and the center of body and mind harmonization. It is the core of selfless impulses, the will to sacrifice for others' welfare.

• The throat is the place of the fifth chakra, which has to do with the ability to discern and communicate. It is the focus of intellectual pursuits and correspondence of greater complexity.

• The third eye, the space between the eyes, is the location of the mind and the sense of individuality. Since it is also the center though which subtle communication takes place, it is also called the "guru chakra."

• Ultimately, the crown of the head belongs to the superconscious state of transcendence of body consciousness. It is the source of the true, universal consciousness.

34. pratibhad va sarvam

Or, all the powers come by themselves in the knowledge that dawn by spontaneous intuition (through a life of purety).

The powers can manifest even when they are not being sought. They may appear spontaneously as the natural result of purity, and as an unselfish, careless mind. This is the best and safest way to attain these powers, since the ego is kept out of the mix.

35. hridaye chittasanvit

The knowledge of the mind-stuff is obtained by samyama on the head.

The fifth and sixth chakras (mental intelligence and seat) may seem more likely to be objects for gaining knowledge of the mind-stuff; instead, Sri Patanjali quotes the heart, hridaya, as the way to gain knowledge of the mind-stuff. For its existence the mind is dependent on the ego, which is better approached through the heart. In this case "heart" refers to the individual's core or "feeling" centre, the place where motives and intent reside.

36..sattvapurushayoratyantasankeernnayoh.pratyayavishesho bhogah pararthatvat svarthasanyamat purushajnanam

The intellect (sattwa) and the Purusha are entirely different, the intellect which exists for the Purusha's sake, while the Purusha exists for its own sake. Not to discern this is the cause of all experiences. Knowledge of the Purusha is obtained by samyama upon this distinction.

Though all of existence is one, single whole, as individuals we only come to know bits and pieces of the entirety of life because we have not encountered the distinction between the Purusha and the intellect. The intellect is finite in nature, and can only learn about the world through the ego's narrow and colored filter.

37..tatah.pratibhashravannavedanadarshasvadavarta jayante

Superphysical hearing, touching, seeing, degusting and smelling arise from this knowledge through spontaneous intuition.

The extrasensory perceptions listed here are a samyama by-product on the distinguishing of intellect and Purusha.

38. te samadhavupasargaa vyutthane siddhayah

These (superphysical senses) are barriers to (nirbija) samadhi but are outsourced siddhis.

These extrasensory powers are expressions of great mental power, but they still exist in the realm of relativity and are obstacles necessary for self-realization to the interiorization of mind. In fact, it is not the powers themselves that are obstacles; it is the attachment to them that is hindering progress. These powers, under the influence of attachment, can tempt egos that are not yet purified of selfishness and become a major obstruction to the experience of the highest samadhi. Since the path to self-realization of each individual is unique in many ways, these powers are not attained by all self-realized individuals. When they do manifest in the enlightened, however, it is a case of the Divine Will working through these great souls to achieve some good.

39. bandhakarannashaithilyat pracharasanvedanach ch chittasya parashariraveshah

Entry into another body is possible by loosening the cause of bondage (to the body) and by knowing the mind-stuff's channels of activity.

Breaking down this sutra phrase by phrase could be helpful.

This refers to the bondage of the mind to the body by loosening the Cause of Bondage (to the Body) It is caused by the ego, born of ignorance (see sutra 2.6, which defines selfishness as the identification of the Seer's power with the instrument of seeing, the body-mind).

Through Understanding the Mind-Stuff's Channels of Action Prachara, translated as "channels," indicates an outgoing or manifestation. It is the knowledge of how the chitta manifests and works within and through a body: the subtle nerve pathways it uses, the mind-stuff relationship with the gross physical body, and an understanding of how the chitta moves at each birth from body to body.

Entering Another (Parasarira) Body Most translators made parasarira as "another's." It continues the sage Vyasa's practice of commenting. But parasarira could be translated as "another." Therefore this sutra could refer either to entering the body of another individual or to attaining an intimate knowledge of the individual's evolutionary journey from birth to birth. The latter interpretation fits with the description of the evolution process discussed in sutras 3.13 to 3.16.

40. udanajayajjalapangkakantakadishvasangg utkrantishch

By mastering the current of the udana nerve (the upward-moving prana), one exerts levitation over water, swamps, thorns, and so on and can leave the body at will.

We've all had the experience of feeling lighter in our bodies—for example, when we are so happy we feel like dancing or jumping for joy. We even use the word uplifted when explaining how good we feel when we hear positive news.

The mind goes inside in deeper states of meditation, and the prana moves upwards, making the body feel light. In reality, for meditators whose feet have fallen asleep it is not an uncom-mon occurrence to have them reawaken without changing their position merely by the ascension of consciousness and a stronger upward movement of the udana prana.

There are several examples of Christianity of saints who levitated naturally. A profound joy in prayer or worship came from that experience. One such example was the Franciscan friar Joseph of Cupertino who, during services, would go into deep ecstatic states, disturbing the service by floating involuntarily around the church's ceiling. While this example does not provide an example of mastery of the udana current, it does demonstrate that similar experiences as those described here can result when it is strongly activated, as in ecstatic states. In advanced yogis cases, however, the udana current may be brought under their conscious control, making the above-mentioned manifestations at will possible.

41. samanajayat prajvalanam

The radiance that surrounds the body comes through mastery over the samana nerve current (the equalizing prana).

Samana prana's function is to maintain equilibrium in the body by transforming food into a cell-usable form and then distinguishing between that and the waste to be eliminated.

The samana prana is rooted in the abdomen, the seat of our digestive "fire." Digestive fire increases in strength and efficacy through samyama on the samana nerve current. The body is growing in fitness and having a healthy glow.

It also associates the fire element with intelligence, specifically as the ability to discern what is harmful and what is beneficial. Fire is associated with discrimination, in the form of light. The transformation and discrimination processes are also carried out on a mental level. The mind has to digest experiences and discriminate between what's useful (suitable for assimilation) and what's useless or harmful (to be eliminated).

By this samyama, the element of fire becomes focused and refined, greatly increasing the mind's discriminative capacity. A special radiance is produced by this, and by what has been said above. This radiance in spiritual artwork might be what we see depicted as halos or auras.

42. shrotrakashayoh sanbandhasanyamad divyan shrotram

Supernormal hearing becomes possible through samyama on the relation between ear and ether.

Ether, akasha, is the sound-associated element; therefore, it has a special relationship to the ear.

One can think of Ether as vacuum. It is the first of all the subtle-elements created. Perhaps we are all familiar with the biblical passage, "The word was in the beginning" (Jn 1.1). There had to be a place to utter it before the word could be pronounced. There is ether in that place.

43..kayakashayoh.sanbandhasanyamal.aghutoolasamapatte shchakashagamanam

Lightness of cotton fiber is attained by samyama on the relationship between body and ether, and thus it becomes possible to travel through the ether.

The body's fundamental building block is Ether (akasha), the subtlest of the elements. When our consciousness can rest on the ether level, our bodies vibrate at their frequency and are able to travel through etheric currents, the waves of ether that permeate creation.

44..bahirakalpita.vrittirmahavideha.tatah.prakashavaranna kshayah

(Virtue of samyama on ether) vritti operation external to the body is no longer (experienced and) assumed. This is the great bodiless that wrecks the veil over the Self's light.

The veil, avarana, is the same word used by Sri Patanjali in sutra 2.52, "As a result (from the practice of pranayama) the veil over the inner light is destroyed." This siddhi is another achievement derived from samyama on the body-space relationship (akasha) when the individual experiences the body's physical boundaries beginning to blend or expand into the infinite ether. The ego-sense begins to experience itself as being unfettered to a specific place.

Our identification with the mind and body is so ingrained that it is no easy task to break. As long as this identification exists, we feel that our thoughts are generated from our body-mind, and so the location of our consciousness is limited to wherever our body resides. Yet we come to experience the mind as omnipresent by samyama on ether, and recognize that it exists and functions both outside the body and within it. This is what is referred to in this sutra as "great bodiless."

45..sthoolasvaroopasookshmanvayarthavattva.samyamadbhootajayah

Samyama gains mastery over the gross and subtle elements concerning their essential nature, similarities, and intent.

Let's look at this sutra in a point-by-point basis.

Gross and Subtle Elements such as all we see, touch, smell, hear and taste are gross elements. The level of the subtle elements is under the level of the gross elements. The subtle is the gross cause.

Essential Nature Subtler than the subtle elements, there is the characteristic essence of a thing: for example, the solidity of a rock, water liquidity, air mobility.

Correlations going deeper; we arrive at the level of the gunas, common to all artifacts. The gunas have an active relationship— a correlation — to the factors set out above.

Purpose lastly; behind all matter, from gross to subtle, is the purpose of matter— the why. Why are there elements at all and why is there a nearly infinite number of objects?

46..tatoanimadipradurbhavah.kayasanpat.taddharmanabhi

ghatashch

From that (mastery over the elements) comes the attainment of anima and other siddhis, body perfection, and the non-obstruction by the power of the elements of body functions.

The eight major siddhis referred to are anima,' to become very small'; mahima,' to become very large;' laghima,' to become very light;' garima,' to become very heavy;' prapati, to reach anywhere; prakamya,' to achieve all of one's desires;' isatva,' the ability to create anything;' and vasitva,' the ability to command and regulate all.'

In its original form, this sutra lists only three siddhis: becoming minute, being bodily perfection, and being free from afflictions caused by Nature's constituents (gunas). The rest of the list, handed down by tradition, is also incorporating references to mental accomplishments.

47. roopalavanyabalavajrasanhananatvani kayasanpat

Beauty, grace, strength, and awe-inspiring hardness are body perfection.

The body perfection described in this and the preceding sutra is the product of the samyama (see sutra 3.45), which brings mastery over the gross and subtle elements.

Yoga practices enhance, refine and harmonize prana functioning in the body. Each cell is charged with potent spiritual vibrations and operates at optimum efficiency.

With this in mind, we might wonder why some great yogis suffered from physical ailments. What we see as physical illnesses are residual karmas that can be manifested from a time before self-realization.

Great experience for yogis that they're not their own body. They will fulfill their obligation to the body by trying different therapies while realizing that the body is made up of Prakriti's elements, and that what is made up of elements will one day melt back into those elements. We recognize that Nature is going to take its inevitable path, and embrace their physical challenges as the will of God. Our minds remain calm.

48..grahannasvaroopasmitanvayarthavattvasanyamad indriyajayah

Samyama gains control over the sense organs on the senses as they interact with the mechanism of perception, the basic essence of the senses, the ego-sense and its meaning.

This sutra resembles 3.45. Instead of turning our attention to matter, here the yogi looks at the process of thinking and how it applies to the ego and the sense organs.

Knowledge causes mastery. The yogi gains control over the senses by knowing the essential nature and purpose of the senses, the role they play in the act of perception, and how they work with and help to maintain the ego-sens.

This samyama can also at least provide some insight into the fact that the Purusha— not the ego-sense operating through the senses — has its own consciousness.

49. tato manojavitvan vikarannabhavah pradhanajayashch

The body develops the power to move as quickly as the mind, the ability to act without the aid of the sensory organs, and total control of the primary cause (Prakriti) from that.

Complete mastery of matter only comes after mastering the organ of the senses and the ego

The Power to Move as fast as the mind this is not a reference to the body's quick transit through space. That's already been discussed. This refers to the mind's ability to function without the impediments imposed by the normal process of perception.

Ability to work without the Help of Sense Organs, the senses is gateway to a great deal of information, and they are used by the mind in the normal course of experiences. But the sense organs are also a limitation, since they can only function within the gross matter relativities. Without them, the adept's mind, having transcended the physical nature of which the senses are a part, can function. This gives rise to the ability to gain instantaneous, intuitive and immediate knowledge. It is an elevated level of clear perception.

50. sattvapurushanyatakhyatimatrasy.sarvabhavadhishthatritvam sarvajnatritvan cha

Through understanding the distinction between sattwa (the pure reflective component of the mind) and the Self, as is omniscience, superiority over all states and modes of life (omnipotence) is achieved.

The subject matter of this sutra is the veil separating the self (ego) from the Self. It is very difficult to distinguish between the Self and its reflection in a perfectly clean and undistorted mirror (pure sattwa, or buddhi). But the benefits are great: it results in mastery, bringing omnipotence and omniscience over all levels of mind and matter. The loosening of Self to the body-mind (which we began discussing in 3.36) is nearly complete. But we still have those pesky samskaras dwelling in the subconscious, able at any moment to sprout and cause mischief.

51 tadvairajnadapi doshabijakshaye kaivalyam

The seed of Self is killed by non-attachment even to that (all these siddhis), and thus follows Kaivalya (Independence).

All siddhis are manifestations of the mind, the result of a focused mind. They exist within creation and are limited; therefore the yogi is still in bondage even when it experiences omnipotence and omniscience. The yogi needs to let go even of the desire to know everything and be all-powerful to attain liberation!

How can we get non-attachment to such seductive experiences? One way is to conduct Ishwara Pranidhana (Ishwara surrender) (see sutras 2.1, 2.32, and 2.45). By Ishwara's worship we can transcend the ego along with any and all limitations that might prevent us from experiencing self-realization.

52. sthanyupanimantrane sanggasmayakarannan punah anishtaprasanggat

The yogi should neither accept nor smile with pride at the admiration of even the celestial beings, as in the undesirable there is the possibility of his being caught again.

Practitioners who have reached a high degree of spiritual maturity also draw other people's attention, whether they are heavenly beings or our earth-bound fellow human beings. The ego loves being stroked and extolled. We are warned that these overtures will not distract us from achieving Self-realization.

In a former life, the celestial beings were unenlightened followers of Yoga.

Their overtures may be motivated by envy of the yogi's progress.

We cannot achieve enlightenment until viveka takes us beyond time and matter. The next four sutras provide a detailed description of that deep degree of discriminatory discernment.

53. kshannatatkramayoh sanyamadavivekajam jnanam

Discriminative knowledge comes about by samyama on single moments in sequence.

The minds appear to underestimate the distinct individuality of the moments as the time blur. It is like watching a film. The illusion we are falling into (and willingly accepting) is that the images are moving, but in reality, what we are seeing is a series of still photos that travel past the projector's light and lens.

It's time we understand change. This samyama unveils time in its most elementary form, as distinct Prakriti waveforms that progressively unfold their inner nature. Self-realization requires the ability to distinguish between change and change (see sutra 2.5, "Ignorance is about the impermanent as permanent...").

54..jatilakshannadeshairanyataanavachchhedat tulyayostatah pratipattih

Thus, the distinct variations in organisms, distinctive markings, and locations between items that are similarly become distinguishable.

Typically, we discern the differences between objects that use one or more of the factors above.

Species we can differentiate, for example; we can tell an apple from an orange quite easily.

Characteristic Marks, if we have two oranges in front of us, we're looking for distinctive marks: Does one have a greenish tinge or a brand label attached to one?

Lastly, if the two objects before us are identical in species and characteristics, then we can distinguish them by their spatial position. One orange is in the fridge while the other is by your side.

But what if we lost all three of those factors? The yogi, whose discernment has grown amazingly, could still discern the difference.

55. tarakan sarvavishayan sarvathavishayam akraman cheti vivekajan jnanam

Nevertheless, intuitive knowledge (which brings liberation) is the transcendent discriminative awareness which simultaneously comprises all objects in all conditions.

That is viveka's zenith. It's "transcendent" because it goes beyond the sutra 3.50 mentioned omniscience. It is a total and perfect experience in all stages, transitions, and conditions— past, current, and future— of the entire created universe at once.

56 sattvapurushayoh shuddhisamye kaivalyam iti

If the calm mind achieves purity equal to that of the Soul, then there is Absoluteness.

This is the natural evolution defined in 3.55 of the discrimination. The mind is back to pure sattwa mode. When the mirror becomes clean and undistorted, it becomes transparent to the Self. It is then that we can understand how we can "be perfect, even as your heavenly father is perfect," in the words of the Lord Jesus (Matthew 5:48)

CHAPTER FOUR
KAIVALYA PADA

1. janmaushadhimantratapahsamadhijah siddhayah

Siddhis are born from past birth practices, or by plants, mantra repetition, asceticism, or samadhi.

Previous Births

God didn't give gifts arbitrarily to people born with siddhis. In previous births, they put forth efforts and are now experiencing the fruits of their labors.

Herbs

There are those who seek a chemical shortcut to spiritual achievements, and have always been.

Mantra Repetition

Although any mantra's concentrated repetition can bring siddhis as a side effect, this sutra is probably referring to the use of mantras intended to produce specific outcomes. Mantras can heal, manifest certain events or objects or bring many more siddhis.

Asceticism

Those who willingly accept suffering and devote themselves to a rigorous course of spiritual practices, gain great mental strength, and may experience siddhis as a result of their disciplines.

Samadhi

The siddhis may also come through the stillness, depth, and purity of the samadhi.

The main teaching is that the goal should not be to siddhis. Siddhis will feed the ego into an impure mind. Nevertheless, if they come as a natural by-product of a selfless, dedicated practice, when it is necessary and useful for them to do so, they will have manifest.

2. jatyantaraparinamah prakrityapoorat

Inflow of nature causes the transformation of one species into another.

Evolutionary force is innate of all beings and objects. It is Prakriti's nature to reveal latent potentialities from birth to regeneration: from embryo to fetus, to birth, maturation, old age, death and then regeneration.

Since jati, translated as "species," also means "birth," this sutra also refers to the gradual evolutionary process occurring for an individual from birth to birth.

3. nimittam aprayojakan prakritinan varannabhedastu tatah kshetrikavat

Incidental events do not directly cause natural evolution; as a farmer they simply remove the obstacles (removes the obstacles in a watercourse running into his field).

The saint waits to manifest within the sinner. The Buddha's heart lies within everybody. Our nature is Divine; to attain enlightenment nothing needs to be added up. Instead, all our efforts are focused on dismantling the barriers that hindered our divinity's speech. As barriers are eliminated, the latent qualities— the potentialities — of each item in Prakriti will naturally express itself. Evolution is, then, a manifestation of every object and being's inherent nature.

The natural selection and survival of the fittest — the theory that competition is the prime mover of evolution — gives an incomplete understanding of the cause of evolution. If competition for food, shelter, and reproduction were to cease, the evolution would continue because of other influences. The light, rain, and soil help the seed grow as a flower of its secret existence. Equally, our interactions with others— good or bad — help bring forth our strengths and weaknesses. Every climate, political, spiritual, astronomical, biological, artistic, and commercial event is an "incidental event," an occurrence that can remove evolutionary barriers.

The subject of evolution continues with a discussion of the creation of individual consciousness over the next three sutras.

4. nirmannachittanyasmitamatrat

Individualized consciousness originates from the primary sense of Self.

Comprehending this sutra is simpler if we look first at the Sanskrit: Nirmana chittani asmita matrat. Nirmana from ma, "to measure, to allocate, to distribute, to make, to create;" chittani, "multiple individual consciousnesses, mind-stuffs;" asmita, "ego-sense;" matrat, "alone, primary, of only." There are two schools of thought about the meaning of this and the two sutras that follow. In the context of evolution, the first school examines these sutras; the second school regards these sutras as an extension of the siddhi discussion.

From an evolutionary point of view, these three sutras are understood to describe the origin of the individual consciousness and its relatedness to the unconditioned consciousness which is the Purusha. In this context, therefore, nirmana chittani is seen as the "individualized mind-stuffs" that evolve from asmita matrat, the "primordial ego" (mahat in philosophy of Sankhya). Asmita matrat is an unparticular "I-am-ness" which makes possible the phenomenon of every individuality.

The second school of thought is inspired by a commentary from the sage Vyasa. His interpretation, based on the assumption that these sutras are an extension of the siddhis debate, for the same terms relies on different shades of meaning. Nirmana chittani is defined as "mind-stuffs that have been artificially created," and asmita matrat refers to the yogi's own ego as the source of those "made" minds. Therefore, these sutras are seen as addressing yogis' desire to actively build other minds in order to accelerate the purging of their past karmas or to increase their ability to serve others.

5. pravrittibhede prayojakam chittam ekam anekesham

Through the individualized minds ' activities may differ, one consciousness is the initiator of all of them.

Chitta ekam, translated as "original mind-stuff," is yet another way of referring to the asmita matrat principle.

With separate "lives" and activities, Asmita matrat creates the appearance of many individual consciousnesses. In truth, behind all the egos there is only one all-encompassing awareness. The Purusha's pure, indivisible consciousness pervades all embodiments of Prakriti

6. tatra dhyanajam anashayam

Of these, what is born for contemplation (the different activities in the individual minds) is without residue.

The residue to which this sutra refers to include subconscious thoughts, samskaras, which drive the mind into relentless action.

Vritti activity leaves impressions — memories — accumulated that dwell in the subconscious mind. Since selfish desires lurk behind most vritti activity, the subconscious accumulations that result are a source of future pain; they nudge the mind towards an endless search for new diversions. Most mental activity left by the samskaras is like a sack of karmic seeds waiting to sprout.

Thoughts arising from meditation can be quite diverse. Meditation impressions promote deeper excursions into equanimity and stillness. As the mind focuses on one thing, the vrittis ' whirling stops. The samskaras left through meditation are purpose-unified; they lead to the transcendence of ignorance. The landscape of the mind is not marred by longings in meditation, but is characterized by an organic movement towards self-realization. These samskaras do not leave any accumulation; they are residue-less.

We are now coming to the final in this series of evolutionary sutras. This time, the emphasis is on karma (cause and effect) and its relation to desires, subconscious impressions, and the evolution of character traits of individuals.

7. karmashuklakrishnnam yoginah trividham itaresham

The yogi's karma is neither white (good) nor black (evil); there are three sorts for others (good, poor, and mixed).

Yogis who have done away with prejudice do not build karma irrespective of whether good or bad. We are Beings of Liberation. Their acts no longer serve to further their evolution, as their efforts have already brought them to the highest state of spirit.

Those who continue to perform their illusory dance in ignorance must face the consequences of the karma that ego-centered actions have created: pleasurable, painful, or mixed.

Similar Sutra: 2.12: "In these obstacles the womb of karmas has its source, and the karmas bear experiences in the births seen (present) or the unseen (future)."

8. tatastadvipakanugunanam evabhivyaktirvasananam

From that (threefold karma) follows the manifestation of only those vasanas (subliminal traits) for which the conditions for producing their fruits are favorable.

To understand this sutra, it will be useful to discuss briefly three principles: Samskaras: Karmasaya subconscious impressions: depository of karmic residue Vasanas: subliminal personality traits, tendencies, and potentialities that form and help maintain habit patterns Samskaras Every thought, word, and deed (whether consciously or unconsciously done) becomes a samskara. Samskaras functions as sublimi-nal activators and constantly propels the conscious mind into further thinking and action.

Karmasaya Without her reaction no action is. All reactions are stored up in the subconscious mind as subtle impressions. The karma receptacle is named karmasaya. The karmasaya contains three kinds of karma: those expressed and exhausted in this birth (prarabdha karma); new karma created during this birth (agami karma); and latent karma waiting to be fulfilled in future births (sancita karma).

A subcategory of samskaras is Vasanas Vasanas. They are subconscious impressions which come together to create a subset of impressions regardless of their order of creation: a "family" of related impressions. Since vasanas induce a person to repeat actions, sometimes they are called subtle desires.

Vasanas shape individual personality traits and habit patterns. They reflect self-identity, established under ignorance (avidya) control. In other words, personality traits can only occur in an atmosphere that embraces the ego-sense and the erroneous belief that we are not the Purusha.

The coming-together of related vasanas is the process which brings forth from karmasaya the karma of this birth (prarabdha karma). In effect, the vasanas are channels through which Prakriti's evolutionary force manifests, expressing itself as the birth of the individual and the experiences it will encounter in that life.

9..jatideshakalavyavahitanam.apyanantaryam smritisanskarayoh ekaroopatvat

Vasanas, though separated by birth, place, or time from their manifestation, have an uninterrupted relationship (to each other and to the individual) because of the seamlessness of subconscious memory and samskaras.

This sutra sounds more complicated than it is. Vasanas— which make up our personality's characteristics — do not necessarily manifest in the order that they were created, but move to the front of the line by their intensity. Their intensity, in turn, is the result of experiences which have a profound and powerful influence on the mind.

While the manifestation of vasanas is not a chronologically ordered process, there is a continuous thread of individuality which links personality lifetimes. This has implications in relation to karma's cause and effect. Every person will face the karmas he or she has created, because of the continuity of individuality. While karmas manifestations can be exchanged by groups (as is the case with all baseball fans in a particular rain-out game), they never move from person to person.

Let's further break that important sutra down.

Vasanas; these are personality traits — tendencies — and have been discussed in detail in the sutra before.

Separated by Birth, Place, or Time (from Their Manifestation)

As mentioned above, vasanas do not manifest in the order in which they are created. Some of the characteristics, habits, and tendencies that appear in this life may have been the source of many incarnations before. Vasanas manifest when certain samskaras reach a "critical mass," when they are strengthened by repeated events, or when a single samskara is powerful enough to gain momentum. It becomes like a whirlpool that draws in similar samskaras, and thus becomes an influential player in creating the personality's subconscious framework.

Have an Uninterrupted Relation

Although the vasanas do not appear in the order of their origin, however they still maintain an unbroken connection to the individual who created them through the samskaras that follow the individual from birth to rebirth.

Samskaras are the thread that links all of our past life experiences together. Even when all conscious thought disappears, the subtle subliminal structure of the mind remains, and the strands of samskaras that have woven around it. This mental subconscious aspect follows us from birth to rebirth to self-realization.

In this phrase, the word "memory" may be a little misleading due to the seamlessness of Subconscious Memory and Samskaras. It may be easier to think of memory as the remnants of action rather than the recollection of people, places, or things. Memories are the subset of samskaras that shapes the habits and traits of personality carried into a given lifetime. In other words, there's a unity in their relationship between subconscious memory and vasanas— a seamlessness.

An analogy will help to clarify this cycle even more. We've all seen films in chronological order that don't tell their story. Not only that, but the line of plot changes local and the focus of characters. But although we temporarily leave behind an aspect of the story, we know that in the end, the plot will tie loose ends together and then bring us to a logical and climaxing conclusion. Vasanas are like the scene that we are watching right now. And just as the script for all the scenes is the storehouse, samskaras is the pool from which vasanas are taken. The screen is Prakriti, the film is our lifetime and the Purusha is the light that illuminates it all. It's just that way with our own lives. All we are (and have been and will be) and all we experience works together to bring us to the realization of Self.

10. tasam anaditvam chashisho nityatvat

Because the desire to live is infinite, vasanas, too, are startless.

The desire to live is a product of our eternal essence, which in itself is life. The compulsion to manifest the Self's infinite, immortal essence is also the force behind the procreative desire. To a large extent, having children fosters a belief that we will somehow live past our physical years. It is one of our everyday links to heaven.

Asishah, translated as "desire to live," can also mean "primordial will." Then we could understand this sutra as referring to God's will, which continually creates from Prakriti's store, and then reabsorbs those manifestations into the unmanifest form. Therefore, the subconscious impressions are also eternal, being a part of Prakriti.

11. hetufalashrayalambanaih sangrihitatvad esham abhave tadabhavah

With these four disappearing, the vasanas, being held together by cause, effect, basis and support, also disappear.

This sutra looks at factors that bind individual vasanas. When we know what keeps vasanas running, we might find a way to break the cause and effect chain reaction that connects us.

The source of all subconscious experiences is ignorance.

Related Sutras: 2.3 and 2.4: Chat about ignorance.

Effect

Our actions bear fruit.

Related Sutra: 2.14: "Karmas bear the fruits of merit and demerit-caused pleasure and pain." Basis Mind, which is the storehouse for all impressions.

Support the existence of external objects stimulating the

mentality to form vrittis.

Now that we know what holds vasanas together, how are we going to make them go missing?

Ignorance is the cause of the continued existence of vasanas and the root of all obstacles; by overcoming ignorance through meditation and samadhi, we overcome the limitations of vasanas (see sutras 2.10 and 2.11, "In their subtle form, these obstacles can be destroyed by resolving them back into their original cause (the ego);" "In the active state, they can be destroyed through meditation").

The next six sutras offer a fascinating glimpse into the nature of the objects of sense, their relation to time, and the fact that they exist independently of the perception of them by an individual.

12. atitanagatan svaroopatostyadhvabhedad

Past and future exist as the essential nature (of Prakriti) for manifesting (perceptible) changes in the properties of an entity.

From its inception, all possible forms of an object are within it. They exist as latent seeds within him. An object's previous forms disappear into the past, and become latent potentials. The future form of an object will be the manifestation of the intrinsic characteristics of an object which express themselves according to the conditions in its environment and the external forces which act upon it. The full-grown oak lies in the acorn, as does the old diseased tree, which is being cut down to make mulch. Yet the seed hides within the mature oak, waiting to show up. The seed holds the essence of the past, its family ancestors and the potentialities of all possible forms within it.

Contemplating this sutra can aid in promoting nonattachment. Our stunning and reliable new car has concealed the rusty, dented jalopy within it, in need of constant repair. Under the influence of time, environment and circumstance it will manifest. Someday, anything new will be old and express different qualities because of its age. And just as only a mature tree can pass its genes on to a new generation, what is aged today is helping to bring forth what is new tomorrow. The message is: it's wise not to hold firmly on to anything. Let Nature take its course and experience the beauty that is inherent in the flow of life.

Related Sutra: 3.55: Describes that phenomenon's direct perception.

13. te vyaktasookshma gunatmanah

Those characteristics, whether manifest or subtle, belong to the nature of the gunas.

The three gunas interact with one another constantly, with the balance between the three always shifting. Thus the object's visible features vary over time.

14. parinamaikatvad vastutattvam

The reality of things lies in the uniformity of the transformation of the gunas.

The "uniformity of the transformation of the gunas" refers to the unique features which follow an object from creation to dissolution. This distinctive feature remains consistent throughout all transformations until it disintegrates naturally into its component parts, or is suddenly and drastically altered by an external agent. All improvements with those unique characteristics remain organized and consistent. A rock unexpectedly doesn't turn into wood. Its rock-ness is a homogeneous quality that follows from mountain to boulder to small pebbles.

Throughout the decades of life in a human body, countless millions of cells are born, function and then die. The liver today is made up of an entirely different set of cells than it was seven years ago. Yet there's still a liver left; your liver. The liver keeps to its liver-ness. The role and purpose remain the same.

Going a step further, assume that the components you absorbed from the food and water you consumed make up your transformed liver. Your liver now is cellular bits of potato, apple, and lettuce. Perhaps your diet has become your body. It happens, of course, to every organ in the body. When cells died away and were replaced, the feeling of your individual identity did not fade away.

What strength gives your body continuity, while keeping its essential character distinct and intact? Why don't you transform into a head of iceberg lettuce after eating salad for ten years, becoming cool, green, and leaflike? From a spiritual perspective, we can say that the purpose is what gives and maintains individuality. Sri

Patanjali teaches that all of Nature (Prakriti) exists for the Seer's (Purusha's) purposes (see sutra 2.21, "The seen exists only for the Seer's sake"). This suggests that everything in creation has a specific intention. And that goal, the object of all things in life, is to "provide the Purusha with experiences for liberation" (see sutra 2.18). Intent is the architecture that remains intact, keeping a being or entity separate through all its physical changes.

15. vastusamye chittabhedat tayorvibhaktah panthah

The perception of even the same object may vary due to differences in different minds.

The differences in perception are due to the peculiarities (the limitations and biases that are based on past experiences) of the different minds ' content.

16. *na cai ka cittatantram vastu tad apramanakam tada kim syat*

Nor does the existence of an object depend upon a single mind, for if it did, what would become of that object when it was not perceived by that mind?

Many philosophy schools believe there is no external truth to the mind of the person. If this were valid, then the original entity would cease to exist when that mind shifted its attention to another object, and would not be perceivable to anyone else. To that philosophical point, Sri Patanjali offers an alternative perspective.

The next ten sutras lead to Self-realization, a state called dharmamegha samadhi, being at the very door. To achieve that, we need to be able to perceive the distinction between the individual mind's limited awareness and the Purusha's unlimited consciousness.

Before going on, revising the groundwork that prepared us for these final steps will be helpful.

• Pada Three dealt with the siddhis: ways of understanding the relationship between matter as well as mind and matter.

• The beginning of Pada Four continued to examine matter through the presentation of the yogic view of evolution, including reincarnation.

• Matter has been described as having a reality (evolutionary life) separate from the mind.

• Evolution was also discussed as it relates to Prakriti's inherent urge to express latent potentials and power

• At a more subtle level, it was seen that the individual mind, the organ of perception, had as its basis the primordial ego, asmita matrat (see sutra 4.4). In the explanation on sutra 1,2 the principle of ego as the basis for individual minds (along with the other two facets of mind, manas, and buddhi) was introduced.

• In the meantime, if we consider our past history as the immediate cause of the conditions of our life and our experiences therein, we will come to a more profound understanding of our lives.

In short, we should have a good working understanding of matter, cause and effect and the nature of mind at this point.

17. taduparagapekshatvat chittasya vastu jnatajnatam

An object is known or unknown regardless of whether the mind gets colored by it or not.

The universe is a series of Prakriti waves which express themselves as names and forms. During their evolution, the names and forms change appearance and then dissolve back into the undifferentiated matter. Such gestures inside Prakriti attract the mind like a snake charmer hypnotizing a cobra through the senses.

Perception happens when an object attracts the mind's focus through the senses. The senses pass these impressions on to the manas (recording the mind's faculty) which then transmit their presence to the buddhi (discriminatory faculty) and ahamkara (the ego that claims the impressions as its own). In other words, experience occurs when the mind gets conditioned by external stimuli. This perception subjectively makes it appear as if the subconscious has its own consciousness. In reality, the Purusha's "borrowed" perspective on the mind is our individual con-science. This is analogous to a mirror that can borrow the sun's light and reflect it into a space. This fundamental misperception— that "own" consciousness of our mind (which is equal to avidya)—is what has stopped us from understanding our True Identity as the Purusha.

Similar sutras: 2.5 and 2.6: the concept of arrogance and selfishness.

18..sada.jnatashchittavrittayastatprabhoh purushasyaparinamitvat

The mind-stuff modifications are always known to the changeless Purusha who is their master.

We discovered in the previous sutra that human awareness depends on input from external sources. Hence it is neither stable nor detailed. This is in stark contrast with the unchanging and limitless Purusha consciousness. The idea here is that mental-stuff improvements are being performed against a backdrop of flat, even, and omnipresent consciousness.

The Sanskrit term translated as "God" is prabhu, which means something first arising in a lineage— a progenitor. This tells us that all forms of thought came after the Purusha or are born there. The Purusha, which is itself unchanging consciousness, is conscious of all the changes the mind-stuff is experiencing.

Mental changes (vrittis) control almost the entire time of the mind, whether it is awake, unconscious or dreaming. Contrast is necessary for perception to occur. For starters, most of us were sitting in a train waiting while it picks up and unloads passengers while another train is next to us, which is not moving. We look out of our window and we catch movement unexpectedly. We're not sure for a couple of moments whether our train or the other is moving.

Whether our train is moving or not, there are two ways to tell. When we feel our bodies squeezed back into our seat or if we look through the windows and see the walls of the train station "running backward" away from us, we perceive the difference of sitting still or moving. We'd perceive that it's our train that pulls away from the station, anyway. Perception in both cases occurs against a contrasting component.

19. na tat svabhasandrishyatvat

The mind-stuff is not self-luminous, because it is the Purusha's object of perception.

The mind is the Purusha's object of perception (drisyatvat, literally, "has a clear nature")

The capacity of consciousness that the mind has is a power that is reflected. It is similar to moonlight which is a reflection of the sun's light. The light reflected off the moon may still help illuminate our planet, but it's not the light it gives.

The next sutra expands that evidence.

20. ekasamaye chobhayanavadharannam

The mind-stuff can't simultaneously perceive both subject and object (which proves it's not self-luminous).

When it perceives objects, the mind-stuff can behave as a subject, or it can be an object of perception itself, but it can't do both at once, which means it is not self-luminous.

I can direct the light of a flashlight on an object or on myself but not on both at the same time. Either the object or my body will be in darkness at any given moment. This is in contrast with the Purusha, which itself is black. The depth of ignorance is never understood.

During daily life it may seem as though the mind (chitta) can be simultaneously self-aware and conscious of an object. For instance, I might be conscious of my frustration with the cold wind nipping my cheeks and the vibrant displays of Christmas I see as I walk downtown, but not at the same time. The subjective sensation of dual consciousness is due to the extraordinary pace at which the mind can move between two thoughts.

21..chittantaradrishye.buddhibuddheratiprasanggah smritisankarashcha

If there is postulation of experience of one mind by another, we would have to presume an endless number of them, and the consequence would be memory uncertainty.

This sutra provides yet another evidence of the mind's unconscious existence. It is kind of a "buck stops here" argument for those who would suggest that there is one aspect of the mind that is specialized in watching while another is going through the different processes of thought.

Let's say one part of our mind testifies to another part of our mind. Which means that when I detect a honeysuckle, there's a part of my mind that records the flora, the aroma, the sniffing and yet another portion of my mind that watches all of this. But we do know that we actually know that. If this is so, if we are conscious that one aspect of the mind is watching another, then there must be another facet of the mind to watch the watcher. Maybe this, too, is real. Mind is an entity which is elusive and enigmatic. Perhaps there is yet another part of the mind that acts as the witness. But we know that we know that again. Is there a different aspect of the mind?

Could that be how perception occurs? Really it's not possible. We would be overwhelmed by an infinite number of parts of mind watching one another— each behaving like a tiny ego. Which "mini-ego" memories would store? So how can we get to those memories? Without memory control, learning or thinking in a coherent?

Logic forces us to avoid some places. That somewhere has to be outside of the thought processes. With the Purusha, we end our search, not as an analyzer, creative thinker, or questioner, but simply as the unchanging, unwavering, unjudgmental witness. Again we are reminded that the consciousness that seems to be the mind's inherent property is but a reflection of the Purusha's unbounded, unconditioned consciousness.

22..chiterapratisankramayastadakarapattau.svabuddhisanvedanam

The function of cognition (buddhi) becomes possible when the Purusha's unchanging consciousness reflects upon the mind-stuff.

This sutra explains the basis of the consciousness of the individual. The Buddhi (also called mahat) is the first of Prakriti's evolutionary manifestations. Being the purest and most subtle aspect of matter, it has a special "nearness" to the Purusha which enables it to clearly reflect the Purusha consciousness. This is what gives buddhi a self-conscious look.

In the world, the countless minds are born from the essence of the one Self. The example below may help to show how this is so.

You just washed your car, and waxed it. A brief thunderstorm roars in shortly afterwards. It's a brief storm, and the sunshine reappears a few minutes later. You notice a lot of droplets of water on the hood of your car. Every drop reflects the whole sun's globe. Even though we can see the sun in every drop, we can't state that the totality of the sun is in that droplet of water. Nor can we say the sun is (limited) affected by reflections in droplets. Yet the light we see and the light we use to experience the sun being mirrored is the sun's light itself. Every mind is like a droplet of water which reflects light. The ego holds the mind together just as the surface tension holds each drop of water together.

23. drashtridrishyoparaktan chittan sarvartham

The mind, in effect, sits and is seen on the Seer's boundary. Although technically part of what is seen, the mind-stuff "borrows" the power of perception from the Self. It is then in a position to have external objects colored or become conscious of them. So we have the ability to comprehend all things.

24. tadasankhyeyavasanachitram api pararthan sanhatyakaritvat

While tainted by countless subliminal characteristics (vasanas), for another's sake (the Purusha) the mind-stuff exists because it can only function in connection with it.

Our daily experiences could lead us to conclude that the mind exists to satisfy desires that our bodies and minds have been given to us for our own sake such as to help us to attain our personal goals. We develop cravings daily and make every effort to fulfill them. We feel better, or more accurately relieved, when we're successful. The whole thing feels so normal that it may seem distant for other purposes to the life of the mind.

While our daily life experience may seem alien, the mind does not exist solely to fulfill personal desires. The mind exists to fulfill a higher purpose than personal gratification, as with everything created within Prakriti. The subconscious exists to serve as the immediate connection to understanding our eternal existence. Like the apple tree that fulfills its ultimate purpose when it reproduces from its source, the seed from which it came, everything in Prakriti finds completion by "returning" to its source: the Purusha That's why the Purusha is referred to as prabhu— the originator — in sutra 4.18.

The ultimate purpose for the existence of the mind— self-realization— can only be experienced at the level of the mind. But the Self's direct experience cannot be achieved by logic, by accumulating information, or by fulfilling desires of sense. Besides these mental functions the mind has a different ability. Like a flawless mirror which perfectly reveals the Sun, a still, clear mind reflects the Self's fullness.

Related Sutras: 2.18: state that Prakriti exists to offer the Purusha both experiences and liberation. The mind is a part of Prakriti; 4.8–4.11: More about vasanas.

25. visheshadarshin aatmabhavabhavanavinivrittih

To one who sees the difference between the mind and the Atman, mental thoughts end forever as Atman does.

This distinction calls for the ability to discern the difference between the original and a prototype copy, that is, the Purusha's undistorted image reflected on the sattwic mind versus the Purusha itself. They look practically the same. We need to overcome the obligations we have to the reflection to make matters more difficult. For lifetime we assumed the reflection is who we are. The identity is impossible to let go of.

"To the seer" refers to a perception deepening or shifting. One can say that Self's misidentification with the mind is the product of sustained one-pointed illusion. The word translated as "thought," bhavana, actually suggests something which is the product of imagination or meditation.

26. tada vivekanimnan kaivalyapragbharan chittam

Then the mind-stuff tends to discriminate and gravitates toward Absoluteness.

This sutra has great beauty and might. The words translated as "gravitates" in Sanskrit are "prak" and "bharam" which means pushing a weight forward, meaning something like a river flowing into the ocean, into its home. If we can take the profound discriminative step described by the previous sutra, if we can discern / experience the distinction between mind and self, we will experience the alluriating whirlpool-like force of the Absolute that leads us to spiritual liberty. The mind is being "moved toward the front," away from ignorance's "weight" and forward to its source. We'll feel the Self's strength lightening up our burden. That power will draw us towards the state of perfect union. You wouldn't be wrong in considering this force as love or grace.

It's not that God is waiting to bestow grace on us for this moment. The grace is always here and there, leading us in countless ways. But it's not always recognizable or feelable. To recognize his presence, our mind has to be still, clear, and free of attachment.

If we feel the pull of the Absolute, is there a practical benefit we obtain? Our consciousness— our network of inner guidance— is infallibly secure, with nearly every motivation being an unconscious nudge that accelerates our path to self-realisation. We will be able to distinguish an incantation from the Absolute as opposed to the ego's call. Next is the perplexing question; how do I know the will of God? Is it going to come to a realization? After years of feeling our way through a dark tunnel, we are now being led by a clear vision of light— a light we envisioned, pursued, and theorized about, but now recognize. There is no doubt about it; we are back home.

27. tachchhidreshu pratyayantarani sanskarebhyah

Owing to past impressions, distracting thoughts may arise in between.

When we forget that we are the Self and fall back with the mind into misidentification, misleading thoughts— born of ignorance — arise again.

Related Sutra: 1.4: "The forms of mental modifications are assumed at other times (the Self appears to be)."

28. hanam esham kleshavaduktam

Related Sutras: Obstacles: 1.30: "Mental distractions are obstacles"; 2.3: "Ignorance, selfishness, attachment, aversion, and clinging to bodily life are the five obstacles." Methods for removing them: 1.27–29: "Mental distractions are obstacles"; 2.3: "Ignorance, selfishness, attachment, aversion, and clinging to bodily life are the five obstacles." Let's also note that back in sutra 1.12, to resolve the pitfalls of vritti operation, we were given the broad-spectrum yogic "pills" of practice and nonattachment. Practice of yoga requires every act that gives the mind steadiness, transparency, and objectivity.

The final six sutras start counting down to the highest spiritual experience.

29. prasankhyanepyakusidasy sarvathavivekakhyater dharmameghah samadhih

The yogi, who does not have self-interest in even the most

exalted states, remains in a state of constant discriminative discernment called samadhi dharmamegha (dharma cloud).

We have already covered a range of different samadhi categories. Dharmamegha samadhi doesn't necessarily represent a separate form. It is more or less a synonym for the samadhi asamprajnata. But it is also a slow-motion, freeze-frame view of asamprajnata samadhi's maturation into full Self-realization.

Before further examining dharmamegha samadhi, let us review the preceding conditions:

• Nirodha was developed to the point where lower levels of samadhi were experienced, leading the yogi to the source of individual perception (see sutra 1.17, samprajnata, or cognitive samadhi).

• The yogi loses interest in seeking or attaching to any and all rewards— spiritual as well as mundane. It represents param vairagya, the ultimate non-attachment state mentioned in sutra 1.16.

• Viveka, the faculty of prejudice, has achieved its highest expression: an unwavering knowledge of the difference between that which changes (Prakriti) and that which is unchanging (Purusha) (see sutra 2.26, which presents viveka as a way of overcoming ignorance).

• The functioning of the gunas has reached its most refined level: purified sattwa has led to omniscience (see sutra 3.50); purified rajas have led to unattached activity (see sutra 4.29); and tamas, cleansed of excessive heaviness, leads to a stable body capable of perfectly relaxed quietness that does not unduly impose its presence on the contemplative mind (see sutras 2.47 and 2.48 on p.

• The tug of the Universal, which started to distinguish the difference between the ego and the Body, is now almost overwhelming. The mind, purified of ignorance, is virtually drawn by the force of a powerful magnet toward union with the Absolute as an iron bar, free of thick, encrusted rust and mud.

That helps us to describe samadhi dharmamegha. The first challenge we face in examining this state is to translate the word "dharma." It is a term brimming with important meanings, most of which fall into one of two categories:

• Virtue, law, duty, purpose of life, and righteousness

• Form, characteristic or function (the word is used this way in sutras 3.13 and 4.12) Moreover, the result is the same irrespective of the interpretation. There is a permanent change in identity from one dependent on the mind-stuff's actions and systems to the pure, unchanging consciousness which is the Purusha.

Raja Yoga's miracle is that training for this state was not a valiant effort to deny or torment the body and mind, but plain, effective practices.

30. tatah kleshakarmanivrittih

All afflictions and Karmas cease from that samadhi.

Dharmamegha samadhi does away with all afflictions and

removes the practitioner from the cause and effect wheel. The yogi becomes a jivanmukta, a liberated being while still in the body; an experience that lies ahead for us all, though we do not know when.

Contrast this sutra to sutra 1.24, wherein Ishwara's virtues include being unaffected by afflictions, acts, or the fruits of actions. Is Sri Patanjali suggesting that at the level of dharmamegha samadhi, we realize that we are identical to Ishwara, the Supreme Purusha in some significant way? Are we really beyond all afflictions: arrogance, selfishness, desire, aversion and bodily attachment? (See paragraph 2.3). Could it be that in fact we are free from all karmic muddle? Are we really this free?

Sure, and even more. We understand this degree of freedom with dharmamegha samadhi because ignorance loses its impact upon our minds.

Related Sutras: 2.3–2.9: klesas (obstacles); 2.10, 2.11, and 2.26: methods for removing klesas; 2.27: "In the final stage, one's wisdom is sevenfold." The last three stages of this sutra describe an experience similar to that discussed here.

31. tada sarvavarannamalapetasy jnanasyaanantyajgyeyam alpam

Then all of knowledge's coverings and impurities are completely removed. What remains to be known is almost nothing, because of the infinity of this knowledge.

Dharmamegha samadhi removes all the impurities that make

knowledge obscure. In this sutra, it should not be mistaken that "intelligence" is information obtained through the senses or conceptualization.

Here "knowledge" stands for the dharmamegha samadhi, the direct intuitive experience. The "infinity of this knowledge" therefore does not refer to an endless expansion of facts but to the reflection of the Purusha — pure unbounded consciousness, the witness of all phenomena— on a pure sattwic mind.

This sutra says that "what remains to be known is almost nothing." The answer to these questions is what remains to be known: what is the awareness experience when it is devoid of content and location (ego) and outside of time? Who am I when the only "I" I now know disappears?

Related Sutra: 3.55: "Intuitive knowledge (which brings liberation) is the transcendent discriminative knowledge which simultaneously comprises all objects in all conditions."

32. tatah kritarthanan parinamakramapari samaptirgunanam

The gunas then terminate their transformation sequence because they have fulfilled their function.

The gunas are like teachers who give us the lessons we need to go further than ignorance. Once we have learned the lessons and passed the examinations, we no longer have to study the same subject again. Our minds are getting free from Nature's constraints.

The Prakriti measure that constituted the human body and mind—which until now had been known as our self-identity, a solid three-dimensional reality — begins to dissolve into the consciousness experience as the one freestanding, unchanging reality. Time and space relativities melt into a cosmic oneness, the Self's perfect, pure awareness.

Related Sutra: 2.18: "The visible is of the nature of the gunas... whose purpose is to give the Purusha both experiences and liberation."

33. kshannapratiyogi parinamaparantanigrarhyah kramah

At the end of their transformations, the sequence (of transformation), and its counterpart, moments in time, can be recognized.

All the efforts the yogi has put into eradicating ignorance is aimed at: the misperception, the misconception that self-identity is confined to the body-mind. This illusion was aided by the ego's fascination with Prakriti's dance, the never-ending play of objects and events that enchant the attention of the mind. It's not so much that the ego is gullible (although it may be and often is); it's rather that Prakriti's show is so convincing. It is a show whose very essence is perfectly designed to trick our senses and cause perceptional errors. (But note that this series is not a cruel practical joke; it is a drama designed to entertain and teach us — to give us the insights we need to achieve self-realization.) For instance, when we look at a twig, our senses interpret it as a continuous piece of matter. Our understanding of the solidity of the twig does not alter even though we know that research has shown that the twig in our hand is mostly vast expanses of empty space interspersed with the minutes of particles that do not necessarily have a material existence.

This sutra explains that transition, which is how we perceive time, is really the shortest measure of time, a set of distinct successive states associated to moments. It's something like the old cartoon flipbooks where a series of sequential sketches in a small book are bound together. The difference between one picture and the next is so slight we may not notice any variation. But when we flip the series in front of our eyes quickly we perceive change. The figures in the cartoon appear to be moving. Every single drawing is a distinct state that flows past our eyes riding moments of time. We experience such powerful illusion each time we go to the movies, this process can be created.

Just as with the cartoon flipbooks, in fact, motion pictures are a series of still images, each slightly different, projected on a screen in rapid succession. It is because in the pictures we experience movement that we can become involved in the story being presented. And we may be happily seduced by the illusion of motion until something happens to interrupt the flow of individual images that move past the light of the projector or transfer our focus from the frame. Whether it's a technical malfunction, a loud sneeze nearby, the inviting aroma of warm popcorn, or an insistent tap on the shoulder of a friend, the result is identical. The "movie world" leaves our attention and is thrown back to us and our environment.

In other words, we are returning to the "real world." Practices of Yoga are meant to bring us to a similar experience regarding Prakriti.

34. purusharthashoonyanan gunanan pratiprasavah kaivalyan, svaroopapratishtha va chitishaktiret

This manifests the ultimate condition of liberation, while the gunas reabsorb themselves into Prakriti, having no more interest in serving the Purusha. And, to look at it from a different angle, the force of consciousness is set in its own existence.

The Self as True Reality is directly experienced as an inescapable truth for the fully realized Yogi. Ignorance faded away. The Purusha's misidentification with the Prakriti has gone forever; the yogi "sees" the true nature of existence, and is completely free from all limitations and pains.

The duty of nature is accomplished, this unselfish mission that our sweet nurse—nature, has put on herself. She kindly takes by the wrist, as it were, the self-forgetting soul and shows it all the encounters in the world, all the forms, taking it higher and higher through the various bodies, until its lost glory returns, and remembers its own existence. Then the good mother goes back the same way she came, for others who have also lost their way in life's trackless desert. Therefore she works without beginning and without end; and so the endless river of souls flows into the ocean of happiness, of self-realization through pleasure and pain, through good and evil.

CONCLUSION

The Yoga Sutras by Patanjali, written centuries ago, is considered as the greatest scriptural text of Indian yogic philosophy. The features of these "threads" are extremely concise, describing important points or strategies, succinctly and often specifically. Such wisdoms were initially oral, made clear, and established by remarks from a teacher directing the pupil.

This meditative obedience of liberation is known as Raja-Royal yoga, or the eight-legged yoga mentioned below:

1. Restraint: nonviolence, not lying, not cheating, not lusting and not attaching

2. Observations: cleanliness, happiness, discipline, self-study, and surrender to God the Supreme

3. Posture, or exercises

4. Breath test

5. Sublimation or retraction from the senses

6. Attention

7. Meditation

8. Concentrate.

Meditation Yoga can be described as union and yoga is also an effort to educate the yogi, the one who practices yoga and how to achieve union with the Supreme consciousness that we call god. Yoga helps us to conquer the idea that our identity as a' person' is a false impression and that our soul is the true us.

The object of these sutras is not to show how to correctly do the asanas, or the best way to sit for meditation. It was believed that before learning the teachings, the students would already have been taught by their instructor the necessary and basics of meditative techniques and asanas.

Such sutras are divided into four sections (padas).

1. Samadhi Pada I: Meditation and Contemplation

2. Sadhana Pada II: Steps to European Union

3. Vibhuti Pada III: Achieved Union and Its Results

4. Kaivalya Pada IV: Enlightenment and Liberty

The Yoga Sutra offers a most excellent cohort for those who would use meditation (dhyana) and other additional yoga activities as a practical spiritual passage to rouse and free themselves. It is important to use Yoga Sutras like any instructional book or industry manual to ensure that the true instructor within is woken up by their own practice. Some translators recommend reading it a little, then practicing it, reading it more, and further practicing, and thus enhancing the process. So we must learn yoga to develop our beliefs and the only way to discover its true nature is to practice it. Our beliefs must lead to "reality," not vice versa.

The open heart discloses that Yoga Sutras as the experiential workbook, it is also mistaken as the point of view of a religious book that could be used to conduct research on the common mind or the intellect. The laboratory is the full world as well as the true nature of consciousness. To find the truth and the instrument of knowledge is to find in this very life the area of knowledge and experience which is independence. Wisdom is by character trans-rational and trans-conceptual; it is also larger than any wave of thought produced, digital notion, as well as technology. A human intellect and its five senses are insufficient to fully map the gyrus spirals of the holographic universe, and Patanjali authenticates everywhere that this holographic truth can be encountered closely if we let go of our bias and predetermined outlooks and false impressions.

According to Patanjali, both knowledge and the intellect (buddhi) come from an ancient source-less intelligence of the universal infinite mind and that is the ever-present pure light inhabiting behind the consciousness often called the param purusha. It is available at all times but only if we choose to search for it. Patanjali says that meditation starts to bear its fruitful results when the traditional linear thought ends and disbands; and the conclusion of the meditation could also be Samadhi (complete incorporation). Here, yoga practice is supposed to be the noun, output and method. The objectless target should be an absolute human true self. Thus the uncultivated samadhi will attain ultimate freedom. Practice alone can help you make yoga to be successful. Only reading in a book about it, and quoting from it or thinking about it won't help. Having said that, when used in conjunction with yoga practice this book still has a significant value.

Thus, Patanjali reiterates the warning against the uselessness of advancing meditation through the intellect; instead recommends that it is important to observe the fruits of yoga such as the acquisition of trans-conceptual knowledge. While emancipation is contingent on throwing away mechanisms of creation and belief systems. Through meditation practice, the initial signs of accomplishment are the emergence of such limits and the immediate awareness of them as obstructions. This will encourage one to look at the sutras from their own perspective and meditative experience in order to understand the sutras at a deeper level. So in a much deeper occurrence and living wisdom of the neutral spirit, one has to rely on the sutras to gain the true and lasting advantage. The aim is not to study the Sutras of Yoga as a conclusion in itself or as an external entity that can be understood, but to use it as a combined effort to practice, and that fused in an authentically poised manner produces knowledge and liberation that patents in our day-to-day existence.

Samadhi Pada (chapter one) is a synopsis of enlightened life (samadhi) composition that describes the yogic system, briefing its critical theory, objectives, and methods. It depicts yoga as the process of conscious assimilation or union of a restrained consciousness functioning within an ego-filled suppressed "self" that has become dishonored, disjointed, or disconnected from its true universal character of mind. The prehistoric root of consciousness, the causal spiritual and universal spirit, the beginning-less shapeless eternal spirit, or the beginning of the all-infusing leads to Self.

In Sanskrit, the mental state is called' citta-vritti' and in the Sutras of Yoga, the mind's changes, twisting, or partiality could be a description of citta-vrtti. It is also the traditional and normal yet artificial state of present-day humanity. It is a blurry and weakened state of consciousness (citta) being disturbed, vague, and troubled structure (Vritti). This then looks like a blowing grass in the wind, a cracked glass pattern, or an insufficient twist that is typically imposed upon the natural unhindered, enormous and extreme scenery of pure unusual consciousness (cit) as normality. Vritti's attachment to the citta produces citta-vrtti; it could also be defined as making patterns of thought that are non-natural, unjust, distorted, counterproductive, and limited, such as a spin that harden the inactive and crude state of endless separation and spiritual self-distancing that distinguishes common double minded thinking. So this path of establishing integration and re-recognition within the samadhi circle is clarified from I.5 all the way to Pada I (nirbija samadhi) ending.

In Sanskrit spiritual practice, sadhana is prominent. For a yogi to switch from a pre-subsisting disconnected, scrappy and dismayed way of living to establishing the links with the fundamental whole where the flight of liberation is known as Yoga Sadhana is granted to the intrinsic living spirit of an être. Comparison of the experience through practice and various other elements is shown in this chapter. In the context of confirmed hypotheses, presumptions, or any of the other Vritti, the numerous other components can be briefly explained as conventionalizations, following clichés, studying politically accepted beliefs. So in this Pada a major focus is given on work. Patanjali also clarifies that true yoga is only for yoga practitioners and not merely for educational purposes.

Made in the USA
Monee, IL
02 December 2020